Vision Loss in an Aging Society

A MULTIDISCIPLINARY PERSPECTIVE

John E. Crews and Frank J. Whittington, *Editors*

AFB PRESS

American Foundation for the Blind

Printed in the United States of America

Library of Congress Cataloging-in-Publication Data

Vision loss in an aging society : a multidisciplinary perspective / John E. Crews, Frank, J. Whittington, editors.
    p. cm.
    Includes bibliographical references and index.
    ISBN **978-0-89128-307-2**
    1. Visually handicapped aged—Government policy—United States.
    2. Visually handicapped aged—Rehabilitation—United States. 3. Visually handicapped aged—Services for—United States. 4. Vision disorders in old age—United States. I. Crews, John E. II. Whittington, Frank J.
    HV 1597.5 .V59 2000
    362.4'1'0846—dc21   99-057908

The mission of the American Foundation for the Blind (AFB) is to enable persons who are blind or visually impaired to achieve equality of access and opportunity that will ensure freedom of choice in their lives.

For Nancy and Kate
—John E. Crews

For Joy
—Frank J. Whittington

Table of Contents

Foreword *Fernando M. Torres-Gil*   *vii*

Introduction   *ix*

Acknowledgments   *xvii*

About
the Contributors   *xix*

PART ONE   **Aging and Vision Loss:
A Statement of the Issues**   **1**

Chapter 1   The Agenda in the Field of Aging
Robert C. Atchley   *3*

Chapter 2   Aging and Vision Loss: A Conceptual
Framework for Policy and Practice
John E. Crews   *21*

Chapter 3   The Knowledge Base for Collaboration
Between the Fields of Aging and Vision
Loss
Alberta L. Orr   *55*

PART TWO   **Multidisciplinary Perspectives
on Aging and Vision Loss**   **83**

Chapter 4   Vision Care for Elderly Individuals:
Innovation and Advancement in Low
Vision Services
Alfred A. Rosenbloom, Jr.   *85*

Chapter 5   Medical Considerations
in the Rehabilitation of Older Persons
Dale C. Strasser   109

Chapter 6   Psychosocial Considerations
in a Rehabilitation Model for Aging
and Vision Services
Bryan J. Kemp   133

Chapter 7   Aging, Vision Rehabilitation, and the Family
Barbara Silverstone   155

Chapter 8   Aging and Disabilities: Collaborative
Practice and Public Policy
Edward F. Ansello   181

Chapter 9   Policy and Funding for Aging
and Vision Rehabilitation Services
Lorraine Lidoff   211

Chapter 10 Directions for Research in Aging
and Vision Rehabilitation
Amy Horowitz and Cynthia Stuen   227

Index   257

Foreword

The demographics of an aging society present a compelling story and a set of immense challenges for all persons, regardless of interests, circumstances, or age. Increases in longevity and the impending doubling of the older population early in the new millennium will make gerontology and geriatrics both "trendy" and vital areas of concern for all Americans. Of the many issues that now spark attention—health and long-term care, housing, transportation, politics, public policy, and research—vision loss and the attendant consequences of losing one's eyesight constitute perhaps one of the least understood set of challenges facing persons as they age. *Vision Loss in an Aging Society: A Multidisciplinary Perspective* puts the complex dimensions of aging and vision loss on the national agenda.

This book makes an important contribution to our understanding of the many facets of experience facing those with eye problems. It does so through a multidisciplinary examination of the elements of professional practice, research, policy, and intervention related to vision loss and vision rehabilitation. No other book brings together top scholars from the fields of aging and disability to weave a tapestry of issues and possible solutions that can provide a body of knowledge through which education, training, research, and practice, as well as public policy, can prepare all of us for the possibility of eye problems as we age.

Vision Loss in an Aging Society is a valuable resource for practitioners, professionals at educational institutions, caregivers, and policy makers. As the population ages and we enjoy the benefits of increased life expectancy, we all have a stake in learning how to manage successfully the potential loss of vision. Few losses cause more fundamental disruptions in the life of an individual than not being able to see properly, yet, with objective information, knowledge, and sensitivity, much can be done to change stereotypes, prevent additional loss or deterioration, and ensure that rehabilitation services and access to eye care are available to those who need them.

Living long and living better are not mutually exclusive if we are prepared for the vicissitudes of old age and if we adjust to the myriad changes that affect us as older persons. The multifaceted impact of vision loss, both as an individual experience and as a public health phenomenon, can be greatly alleviated with the lessons to be learned through the ground-breaking collection of analyses and treatises presented in this book.

Fernando M. Torres-Gil
Former Assistant Secretary for Aging
U.S. Department of Health and Human Services
Director
University of California Center
for Policy Research on Aging

Introduction

A great structural change is occurring in the United States. For most of this country's history, the cohort distribution of the population resembled a triangle, with large numbers of young people at the base, fewer numbers of working-aged individuals in the middle, and a relatively small number of older persons at the apex. In the early decades of the 21st century the distribution of the population will resemble more of a rectangle, as the population of older, middle-aged, and young people becomes approximately evenly distributed. This change in the size of various population segments has implications far beyond its abstract geometric shape, and some effects of the shift from a youthful to aging population are already evident in the marketplace. Clothing is cut a little fuller, architects and builders are designing homes for empty nesters, and evening news commercials are dominated by treatments for late-middle-age maladies. Hallway conversations among baby boomers occasionally focus on concerns about financing retirement and caregiving for older parents. Other changes reflecting the aging of the population are yet to come, and we can only imagine how we, individually and as a society, will respond.

Much discussion in the area of public policy and aging has focused on the anticipated increases in the overall older population and more recently on increases in the incidence of age-related diseases and disabilities. Conditions such as arthritis and Alzheimer's disease have moved forward as public health and public policy issues. As advocates and researchers assert that greater numbers of older people will experience age-related disabilities, the numbers projected for individual impairments begin to sound alike, as we hear that the number of persons experiencing this disease or that illness will double in the coming decades.

Curiously absent from these public policy debates is a discussion of the situation defined by more than three million older people now experiencing visual impairment, whose numbers are expected to swell dramatically over the next two decades. It is puzzling that although most people fear vision loss as much as they do cancer or AIDS, the topic of blindness rarely surfaces in the press or popular literature. Occasionally, we will hear of medical advancements in the treatment of eye diseases, or we see an individual or family that has "overcome" a disability. Sometimes, these stories respect and honor the human experience of disability, but too often, they slip into tawdry portrayals of victimization or heroism. Much of the reality of aging and vision loss is defined by individuals and families struggling quietly, often very much alone, doing the best they can to accommodate themselves to the challenges presented by the powerful combination of advancing age and declining vision.

Often the declines experienced in visual acuity by individuals are gradual, and therefore, interpreted in some way as "normal." One may stop driving and rely on others for transportation. Declining vision may make it increasingly difficult to read the newspaper, and therefore, one gleans the news from the larger type used to announce headlines. Walking about may become increasingly difficult because obstacles may threaten falls, and eating out may no longer be a pleasure because one cannot read a menu or distinguish the food on a plate.

It is not that "nothing can be done" in such cases. Effective interventions are available for many circumstances, such as those provided by low vision rehabilitation professionals, who can prescribe optical aids to enhance residual vision, or by orientation and mobility instructors, who can generally teach older people how to travel in relatively unfamiliar environments and to use public transportation. Rehabilitation teachers can provide instruction in meal preparation, methods of communication, and strategies for organizing the home. And many social workers and counselors successfully work with older individuals, families, and groups of consumers to help them adjust to new circumstances. Often, too, larger groups of older people gather together in peer support networks to share strategies, frustrations, and successes. These interventions define a robust array of rehabilitation services helpful to older people. But according to a 1995 study conducted by Lighthouse International in New York City, only 1 percent of people surveyed were aware of or availed themselves of rehabilitation services. In many respects, these figures should not be surprising. Although few people know about services and fewer still take advantage of them, the reality is that there is a great paucity of services available to older individuals. The system of community agencies in this country is largely underfunded and unable to respond to the rehabilitation needs of older persons, and although the federal government has attempted to assert a leadership role, a modest funding of about 11 million dollars is inadequate for the millions of people whose needs, as well as numbers, are expected to strain current resources. Moreover, rehabilitation services by and large are not reimbursed through third party payments. The net result is that this country has a rapidly increasing population of older people experiencing vision loss but virtually no system in place to respond to this very serious and pressing need.

This situation should be characterized as a national scandal and a tragedy of immense proportion. It is not. Vision loss among the elderly too often is viewed as a personal tragedy, not a public responsibility requiring a broad, concerted response. Aging and vision loss represent one of the great unaddressed social issues of contemporary America.

Ten authors have joined the editors of this project to increase the level of understanding of the scope of complexities entailed by aging and vision loss and to propose strategies to respond to this complex experience. We have by design involved contributors who represent research, policy, and clinical perspectives from the aging community because we want readers from the field of aging to be drawn to this book to learn more about people who are both older and visually impaired. Similarly, we believe it essential that readers from the vision rehabilitation community become more attuned to the perspective that work in the area of aging brings.

The scholars whom we have chosen have not disappointed us. Like artisans detailing the warp and woof of a fine carpet, they have sounded themes to be woven together from the differing perspectives that they represent. Themes related to the design of interventions, impact of demographic forces, anxieties of caregiving, and lack of concerted policy and rigorous research embrace in this one volume the complexity of the experience defined by aging and vision loss. The authors represent some of the brightest and most perceptive thinkers in the fields of aging and vision rehabilitation. Robert Atchley, a highly respected scholar in aging, observes that the aging community has done little to understand or respond to the needs of older people who experience vision loss. He notes that many of the issues that define the "aging agenda"—health care, housing, and economic security—although benefitting all older people, have not directly responded to the particular rehabilitation needs of older people who have lost vision. He proposes a "common ground" that forces us to look anew at a particular group of older people who should be incorporated into the routine of the aging services network.

Alberta Orr draws on her considerable experience in aging and vision rehabilitation to discuss the need for a common body of knowledge on aging and vision loss. Her target audience focuses principally on gerontologists who understand aging well, but are less familiar with vision loss. She summarizes key historical events that have helped to shape services for older people with vision impairment and also reviews the causes of vision problems that affect most older people. By defining a core knowledge base, she prepares professionals in the field of aging to better serve people who are visually impaired.

Al Rosenbloom, the director of low vision services at the Chicago Lighthouse for People Who Are Blind or Visually Impaired, provides a scholar-practitioner point of view as he reviews both normal and abnormal changes to the eye, the role of low vision in rehabilitation, and research needs in low vision optometry. Dale Strasser, a physician trained in both aging and rehabilitation, helps to clarify physical changes and medical issues that face all older people, and he gives particular attention to those who experience vision impairment. Normal and abnormal changes to the body associated with aging can be exacerbated or accelerated because of vision loss. Falls and fear of falling, a reasonable concern for all older people, for example, become particularly problematic when vision loss creates difficulty in identifying trip hazards.

Bryan Kemp's work spans well over two decades, and 10 years ago he coedited *Geriatric Rehabilitation,* proposing that older people could benefit from rehabilitation interventions, a fairly novel idea at the time. In his chapter, he explores the complex psychosocial dimensions of older individuals and families as they come to terms with vision loss. He notes the particular characteristics of older people in rehabilitation, and he defines the complex confluence of psychological stress and family dynamics in achieving quality of life outcomes. Kemp observes the resilience of individuals to achieve what he calls "valued activities."

Barbara Silverstone, the director of Lighthouse International, draws on her clinical and research experience in aging and the family to describe the largely unexplored arena of social support among older people who are visually impaired. She recognizes the role of the family in rehabilitation, a logical but ignored concern, and she successfully characterizes what it is that is different about aging and vision loss as that impairment is related to other age-related disabilities.

Ed Ansello and Lorraine Lidoff tackle the thorny problems of the public policies that have emerged about aging, disability, and vision loss. Ansello provides a broad frame within which the evolution of public policy and disability are defined and the interface of those policies is considered with emergent aging concerns. The intersection and interweaving of these two broad domains—aging and vision loss—seem logical and predictable, but that has not been the history. Lorraine Lidoff addresses the specific policies that surround funding for national rehabilitation services and obtaining third-party payments for rehabilitation interventions. These two authors reveal to us that older people experiencing vision loss are devalued in multiple ways that have hampered the evolution of policies that other older people take for granted.

Amy Horowitz and Cynthia Stuen, researchers and analysts with a depth of experience, define central issues related to conducting research in aging and vision loss. The concerns they identify are raised throughout this book, and among other things, include the lack of clarity about numbers. Most studies, for example, regarding aging and vision loss are comprised of small sample, cross sectional data; clearly population-based samples that provide longitudinal data are more powerful and are badly needed. In addition, the issues of social support; peer supports; comorbidities; adaptation strategies; and age, ethnic, and gender differences all require attention. Horowitz and Stuen insightfully define these problems and reveal potential strategies for better understanding them.

The magnitude of this project may prompt some observers to ask why this book on aging and vision impairment was written. We would like to suggest four reasons:

First, there is a small, but increasing, knowledge base describing the dimensions of aging and vision impairment. A review of the literature reveals this remarkable paucity of information. Horowitz and Stuen cite the work of Rosenbloom and Goodrich, noting that there are twice as many citations regarding children as there are older adults, whereas older people comprise by far the largest proportion of the visually impaired population. This book is, therefore, an effort to increase our knowledge.

The second purpose for writing this book is to capture the *complexity* of this very human, often very difficult experience of vision loss. It is too easy, especially in our rather ageist culture, to assume that vision loss among people who are older is a unidimensional experience. It is not, of course. Vision loss among older people represents something of an intersection between the experience of vision loss and the total life experiences and resources that the individual brings. People who are resilient, resourceful, good problem solvers, and who have deep financial and family resources will probably have a better time of it than people who do not have those characteristics. This is not to imply that vision loss is "easier" for some than others, but we do want to suggest that there is great variability in human experience.

The third goal of this book is to influence public policy decisions surrounding this issue. Aging and vision loss constitute a grave public policy concern and one that deserves serious attention. People who are older and experience vision problems deserve, in our view, service that is as comprehensive, rigorous, and well funded as that available to older people who, for example, experience a stroke. We are far from parity in terms of rehabilitation services for people who are older and visually impaired.

The fourth goal is to "honor" the experience of individuals who deal with vision loss. The onset of vision loss is a life defining event. No one—family, physician, or service provider—should underestimate the profound effect of this event on the individual. The more people understand aging and vision loss, the more sensitive they are likely to become as they perform their various roles, and therefore, the more effective they are likely to be.

In conclusion, the perspectives and skills of many talented practitioners have been brought to bear on a topic that will overtake our society. It should present the beginning of a conversation that will result in thoughtful planning, concerted action, improved services, and heightened understanding.

Acknowledgments

As with any major undertaking, we need to thank a number of people, because completion of this project would never have occurred without their support. Therefore, I wish to thank Elton Moore at the Rehabilitation Research and Training Center (RRTC) on Blindness and Low Vision at Mississippi State University. Much of the work for this book was completed while I was Research Director at the RRTC. Elton and my colleagues there were most supportive of this project. In addition, I wish to acknowledge Don Lollar and my colleagues at the Centers for Disease Control and Prevention who provided encouragement during the final stages of this undertaking. Nearly 25 years ago, Dr. Ruth Kaarlela encouraged me and others to study aging and vision loss. Ruth was a pioneer and recognized the importance of an emerging field before anyone championed the cause. I wish to recognize her powerful influence. Moreover, I wish to thank the hundreds of people who are older who I have had the opportunity to serve in the years that I worked for the Michigan Commission for the Blind. I learned far more from them than they ever learned from me, and their lives are a testimony to the strength, courage, and resilience that this book attempts to honor. Thanks, too, to Natalie Hilzen and Sharon Shively of AFB Press. Several years ago Natalie asked me to write a book for AFB, and I told her that there wasn't a book in me. She found that book and provided valuable guidance each step of the way. Finally, I wish to acknowledge my wife, Nancy, who consistently provided insight and perspective that touches every page of this book just as she touches every day of my life, and my daughter, Kate, who by her example inspires me to do my best work.

John E. Crews

My acknowledgments are few but sincere. First, I thank my coeditor, John Crews, for inviting me to share the work and the opportunity to learn that have accompanied the editing of this book. I brought some knowledge of aging and editorial skills to the project, but the field of vision loss and aging is primarily John's, and he is one of a handful of such experts around the country. Without John's guidance, insight, and understanding, I could not have learned enough to accomplish this formidable task.

In addition, I must acknowledge the immense support and encouragement I receive daily from my colleagues and friends in the Gerontology Center at Georgia State: Mary Ball, Mary MacKinnon, Sharon King, Cynthia Griffith, and Carole Hollingsworth are the kind of coworkers we all hope for and highly value, and it is their generous help and support that has enabled me to complete this book. For this and many other things, I am much in their debt.

I also would like to thank Richard Long, of Western Michigan University, who first raised my awareness of vision problems in old age and began my instruction in this area. In addition, Natalie Hilzen and Sharon Shively of AFB Press have been wonderful editors and a pleasure to work with. Their suggestions have not only improved this book but have taught me much about producing good scholarship.

Finally, I want to thank my wife, Joy, for the love, the energy, and the fun she brings to my life. I dedicate not only this book but all my work to her.

Frank J. Whittington

About the Contributors

John E. Crews, D.P.A., is a health scientist in the Office on Disability and Health of the Centers for Disease Control and Prevention in Atlanta, Georgia, and clinical assistant professor, Emory University School of Medicine, Atlanta, Georgia. Dr. Crews is the author of 40 publications on aging and vision loss. His previous positions include research director, Rehabilitation Research and Training Center on Blindness and Low Vision, Mississippi State University in Starkville, Mississippi; and executive director, Governor's Council on Developmental Disabilities, Atlanta, Georgia.

Frank J. Whittington, Ph.D., is director, Gerontology Center and professor, Department of Sociology, Georgia State University in Atlanta, Georgia; he is also adjunct assistant professor, School of Medicine, Emory University, Atlanta, Georgia; and research health scientist, Rehabilitation Research and Development Center on Aging, Veterans Administration Medical Center, Atlanta, Georgia. Dr. Whittington is the author of more than 50 publications related to aging. His previous positions include senior research policy advisor, Task Force on Aging Research, National Institutes of Health in Washington, DC.

Chapter Authors

Edward F. Ansello, Ph.D., is director, Virginia Center of Aging, and professor, Department of Gerontology, at the Virginia Commonwealth University in Richmond, Virginia.

Robert C. Atchley, Ph.D., is professor and chair, Department of Gerontology, at Naropa University in Boulder, Colorado.

Amy Horowitz, D.S.W., is senior vice president for research and evaluation and director, Arlene R. Gordon Research Institute at Lighthouse International in New York City.

Bryan J. Kemp, Ph.D., is director, Rehabilitation Research and Training Centers on Aging with a Disability, and Aging with Spinal Cord Injury; director, Gerontology Programs at the Rancho Los Amigos National Rehabilitation Center in Downey, California; and clinical professor of family medicine, psychiatry, and behavioral sciences at the University of Southern California in Los Angeles.

Lorraine Lidoff, M.A., is director of the National Vision Rehabilitation Cooperative at Lighthouse International in New York City.

Alberta L. Orr, M.S.W., is chair of the National Aging Program of the American Foundation for the Blind in New York City.

Alfred A. Rosenbloom, Jr., O.D., is director of Low Vision Services at the Chicago Lighthouse for People Who Are Blind or Visually Impaired.

Barbara Silverstone, D.S.W., is president and chief executive officer of Lighthouse International in New York City.

Dale C. Strasser, M.D., is associate professor and chair, Department of Rehabilitation Medicine, Emory University School of Medicine in Atlanta, Georgia, and research health scientist at the Atlanta VA Medical Center.

Cynthia Stuen, D.S.W., is senior vice president for education and director of the National Center of Vision and Aging at Lighthouse International in New York City.

P A R T O N E

Aging
and Vision Loss:
A Statement
of the Issues

CHAPTER 1

The Agenda in the Field of Aging

Robert C. Atchley

Despite the availability of a general literature on vision and aging (Atchley, 2000; Kline & Scialfa, 1996; Scheiber, 1992), the field of aging has tended to address issues related to blindness and visual impairment in isolation, not as matters vitally connected to key concepts in that field such as productive aging, active life expectancy, or even dependency. Although vision problems and activity limitation stemming from vision problems steadily increase in prevalence as population birth cohorts pass age 50 (Horowitz, 1994; Scheiber, 1992), the field of aging has not placed a high priority on understanding age-related patterns in vision or in the epidemiology of visual conditions such as glaucoma, diabetic retinopathy, macular degeneration, or cataract. In addition, the field of aging has not considered in any depth how vision-related concerns articulate with other issues that require prevention, rehabilitation, and compensation by aging individuals.

This chapter presents an overview of the policy agenda of the field of aging and the issues driving its advocacy, research, and program priorities. The field of aging is used here to refer to a broad combination of academic gerontologists; government agency staff, service agency staff, and personnel who primarily serve an older client population; advocates for social policy concerns affecting elders; and policymakers who make and implement laws and regulations governing funding and operation of programs serving elders. This chapter also examines trends in the society at large that are changing the agenda in the field of aging and suggests likely new emphases for the near future. Finally, it considers how vision-related issues, especially as perceived by the vision and blindness field, could be articulated with the agenda of social gerontology.

FACTORS DRIVING THE AGENDA OF THE FIELD OF AGING

The growing size and diversity of the aging population, the legacy of Great Society liberalism, the intransigence of social problems such as low income for significant population segments within the aging population, and socioeconomic political forces of change are all combining to reshape the agenda and priorities of the field of aging. No one set of organizations, constituencies, or issues dominates the field; instead, the agenda of the field of aging evolves out of the actions and concerns of thousands of people. People who directly experience aging constitute a broad base of concern with respect to an enormous variety of issues, and vision problems often are seen as being of minor importance or at least as affecting a relatively small proportion of the aging population. Advocates for people who are aging seldom focus on problems stemming from visual changes associated with aging. Service providers usually focus on finding more resources to meet needs that are already well documented, and little energy remains to ponder new areas of need. Researchers need support to investigate the many unanswered questions about aging, but here, too, relatively little interest in vision is apparent. For example, compared to the magnitude of funding provided for research on memory or Alzheimer's disease, the resources devoted to eye research, vision rehabilitation, blindness prevention, or adaptation to low vision, a term commonly used to refer to visual impairment that cannot be corrected and is severe enough to interfere with daily activity, are modest indeed. Professional organizations and institutions of higher education need public support to provide education and training for the large numbers of personnel that will be required as service providers in the field of aging. But the focus is increasingly on personal care for aging people with impairments in activities of daily living, without a clear understanding of the links between age-linked changes in vision and such impairments.

Some people in the field of aging genuinely want to be inclusive, to be receptive to new ideas or concerns. Others resist new agenda items or alliances with other fields because they see them as threats to their hard-won gains in public policy support and program development. Some believe that policy and practice issues of chronic disease and disability should be age irrelevant (Neugarten, 1982); whereas others believe that older people usually are shortchanged when programs are age integrated. There is more research support for the latter view (Pynoos & Parrott, 1996; Spore and Atchley, 1990). Accordingly, the literature about service delivery in the field of aging almost always starts with a presumption that services will be exclusively designed for and targeted to the older population.

THE CHANGING OLDER POPULATION

Of the factors reshaping policy in the field of aging, the increasing size and diversity of the aging population are of primary significance. If the older population is defined as those who are age 65 or older, then the older population is projected to grow rapidly in both numbers and diversity over the next five decades. Although this situation is often mentioned, most people have difficulty conceiving of the enormity of these impending changes. According to population projections from the Bureau of the Census (which have usually underestimated actual growth in the older population), most of the growth in the older population will be concentrated in people of the oldest ages, in whom vision problems and issues are most likely to occur (U. S. Bureau of the Census, 1992). For example, between the years 2000 and 2050, the population of individuals age 85 and older is expected to grow from 3.1 million to 26.1 million. Blindness, low vision, and visual impairment are very common conditions in persons past age 75. For example, Kahn et al. (1977) found an 18 percent prevalence of cataract for those age 65 to 74 compared with a 46 percent prevalence for those 75 to 84. The aging of the older population also will increase the proportion of individuals coping with other forms of disability. For example, at age 85 to 89, about 43 percent of elders have two or more impairments in activities of daily living (ADL); but by age 95 and over, almost three-fourths of people have two or more ADL impairments (Mehdizadeh, Kunkel, & Appelbaum, 1996). It is not known what proportion of ADL impairment in the most elderly of older people can be prevented or compensated for by interventions designed to prevent or offset visual impairment. However, Horowitz (1994) found that about one-fourth of the population in nursing homes had visual impairments that contributed to their ADL dependency, and she also found that vision status was an independent and significant predictor of ADL dependency. Research is needed that can establish age-specific relationships between vision issues and disability for detailed age–sex categories in the older population, particularly among the oldest-old.

If adulthood is considered as starting somewhere around age 20 and middle age as ending around age 60, then the older adult population, with an age span from 60 to 110 or so years, has an age range larger than young and middle adulthood combined. Which is more different, a 50-year-old compared with a 20-year-old, or a 60-year-old compared with a 90-year-old? With age ranges this large, physical, mental, and social individuation can produce pronounced differences, and discussing what is "typical" of various broad age categories becomes increasingly meaningless. By itself, the growing age diversity caused by the increased proportions in the oldest categories within the older population will represent a challenge for programs aimed at the older population as a whole, because as populations become more complex, they become more difficult to describe and summarize. The increased diversity of the older population will come not only from a larger proportion of people in the very oldest age categories but also from the growing prevalence of couples within the young–old population, persons of Hispanic descent becoming the largest minority population, and a growing economic diversity within the older population.

Many of the current programs and services for elders presume that the older population in need consists primarily of widowed women. Although this presumption will remain true for women over age 80, for the younger age cohorts in the older population the narrowing gender gap in life expectancy will mean that a larger proportion of couples will survive into their late 70s or longer. This change will have important implications for family caregiving because spouses are typically the first people called on to provide long-term care in the home. However, research has shown that caregivers who are older spouses need formal service providers who will work together with them from the beginning to prevent the caregivers from becoming exhausted and dependent themselves (Hoyert & Seltzer, 1992).

Today, the African American population is the largest minority in the older population, but by 2050, the Hispanic population is expected to be the largest minority. Differences in language and culture between Hispanic elders and the general older population will represent a growing challenge to the field of aging. This trend also has important implications for the vision and blindness systems because the Hispanic older population has a higher prevalence of chronic diseases with visual complications (Markides, 1989).

In terms of financial resources, the older population will also become increasingly diverse. This growing dispersion of income within the older population will result from both the aging of the older population and significant changes in the structure and adequacy of retirement income systems. Pension income seldom keeps up with inflation, even when pensions are indexed, because inflation does not take into account increases in beginning wages. As a result, retirement income that seemed adequate at the point of retirement can steadily become less adequate relative to the resources available to young and middle-aged members of the labor force. This disparity is especially likely to reach problem proportions for those who are age 85 or older.

Changes in the structure of employment and pensions have led many researchers to expect that by 2050 many retirees will have less adequate retirement incomes compared with those who retired in the 1980s. This negative view is based on several trends: (1) growing concerns about the staying power of Social Security; (2) a decline in the proportion of workers covered by employer pensions; and (3) a decline in defined-benefit pensions and an increase in defined-contribution pensions.

In my opinion, Social Security will continue to provide a base of retirement income in a manner not very different from today. However, many who rely on employer pensions may encounter problems. As career employment with a single employer becomes less common for individual workers, portable defined-contribution plans become more attractive, all other things being equal. But employers have not only moved away from defined-benefit plans, they have also moved away from making substantial contributions to employer pension plans, especially defined-contribution plans. As a result, the amount being invested in defined-contribution pension plans is substantially less than required to provide the necessary retirement income needed to supplement Social Security and produce a retirement income that will allow retirees to preserve their customary lifestyles. The greater the extent to which employer pension plans rely on voluntary contributions by employees, the greater the underfunding of such pension plans tends to be. In combination, these trends in retirement income financing will increase the disparity between an increasingly smaller proportion of financial "haves" in the older population and an increasingly larger proportion of financial "have nots." Thus, a growing proportion of elders will have difficulty finding the resources to pay for their own services or to pay larger premiums and co-payments required by Medicare or private health insurance.

THE LEGACY OF LIBERALISM

Much of the current public policy agenda in the field of aging grew out of the national climate of collective response to social problems that flourished during the Kennedy, Johnson, and early Nixon administrations. In the 1950s the United States was very affluent, but amidst that affluence, grinding poverty, inadequate health care, and substandard housing existed on a large scale among the nation's elders as well as within the nation's minority groups. The spirit of the Civil Rights movement, with its emphasis on gaining a fair share of the nation's prosperity, was a large part of the foundation upon which the field of aging was built.

The current policy agenda closely parallels the manifesto outlined in Title I of the Older Americans Act of 1965 that challenged the nation to provide its elders with income security; access to much-needed physical and mental health care; suitable housing; rehabilitative services for those in institutional care; continued opportunities for employment without age discrimination; dignified retirement; continued opportunities to participate in the civic, cultural, and recreational life of communities; access to community services such as transportation and multipurpose senior centers; research aimed at sustaining and improving health and happiness in later life; and the right to self-determination in their life choices. This extraordinarily broad agenda was mainly symbolic, but it conceptually set the older population apart as an especially deserving population category that needs to be given high priority in terms of access to national resources.

Those who have worked in the field of aging during the past 25 years experienced the exuberant optimism of the early 1970s, when it appeared that steady progress would continue toward achieving the agenda of the field of aging that had been codified in Title I of the Older Americans Act. They also experienced the growing pains within the field as it grew larger and more complex. As resources for aging services leveled off in the 1980s, turf battles developed between those who wanted to continue expansion of early programs and those who saw the need for new and different kinds of programs. For example, multipurpose senior centers were required to shift their emphasis from programming for all older Americans to focusing more of their resources on programs for economically and socially disadvantaged elders. The rapidly growing need for home and community-based long-term personal care and homemaker services put intense pressure on all funding sources in the field of aging, often sharply narrowing the segments of the older population whose needs could be addressed.

If progress with respect to achieving the agenda for older Americans is viewed objectively, it is clear that enormous strides have been made. Social Security reforms of the early 1970s, the creation of Supplemental Security Income (SSI) as a genuinely national program of income support for elders in poverty, Medicare, Medicaid, federally subsidized housing for low-income older Americans, various home- and community-based care initiatives, and countless other program and service developments created a loosely structured system that serves the needs of a large majority of the older population. On the other hand, millions of older Americans still cannot meet their most basic needs for adequate income, housing, or care. More than a fourth of the older population still have incomes near or below the poverty level. The federal government has all but abandoned its commitment to low-rent housing for elders living at or below the poverty level, and the housing supply for near-poor elders is shrinking. States routinely close off access to Medicaid-funded health services once current funding limits are reached. For example, in one state, no new Medicaid clients can be served after March or April of each fiscal year unless a current benefit recipient leaves the program. Thousands of elders who qualify are thus left on waiting lists, not for services but for funding. But although many of the distressing conditions that gave rise to the field of aging services still remain, albeit in smaller proportions, the public and its policymakers have tired of hearing about these problems, which seem so intractable.

The lack of Medicare coverage for refractions and corrective eyeglasses represents a major gap in access to needed care, but to advocate for expanded coverage, better estimates of the magnitude of the problems caused by lack of coverage are needed. In addition, as will be discussed later, the funding crisis in Medicare means that expanding Medicare to cover vision services would be very difficult.

The rapid rate of health care inflation was not caused by the aging of the population; however, the fact that older Americans had access to Medicare and poor elders had access to Medicaid made the older population convenient scapegoats for a health system that was financially out of control. The goal of universal access to health care for elders remains, but policymakers have shifted from believing that efficient management of care can minimize costs to believing that only the direct management of costs will work and that currently accessible health care is all the public is willing to pay for. (If all members of the public had access to health care only by lottery, it might rapidly become evident that health care was more affordable than had previously been thought!)

The result has been a rush to "managed care," which usually is not as concerned with managing care or providing high-quality care as with containing the costs of care. The early research evaluations of managed care in the field of aging have not been encouraging about the adequacy of the care provided through this mechanism (Newcomer, Harrington, Manton, & Lynch, 1995; Branch, Coulam, & Zimmerman, 1995), which means that despite increasing federal, state, local, and private health care expenditures, access and quality of care seem to be eroding for elders as well as for most other segments of the population.

Faced with an avalanche of need for health and long-term care when the baby-boom cohorts enter later old age (around the year 2030), the agenda in the field of aging in recent years has placed emphasis on developing as many long-term care options as possible as quickly as possible, while at the same time maintaining a high quality of service and protecting care recipients from abuse and exploitation. Alongside the development of long-term care service options has come a new and sometimes conflicting agenda item of increasing clients' authority to direct their own care (Scala & Mayberry, 1997). A review of the names of current journals in social gerontology and the titles of articles within those journals quickly reveals the great extent to which long-term care issues have come to dominate the field of aging.

SOCIAL TRENDS INFLUENCING THE AGENDA IN AGING

Several trends in the national consciousness have important implications for the future, both in the field of aging and in vision and blindness systems:

- ◆ Concerns about rates of economic growth
- ◆ Eroded confidence in government

- ◆ Preoccupation with so-called entitlements and their effect on the federal budget
- ◆ The decline of the middle class
- ◆ Hopelessness in the face of the growing population of elders in blindness systems

Economic Growth

Despite steady increases in economic growth since 1992, many policy-makers remain skeptical about the nation's capacity to sustain the economic growth required to cope with the needs of an aging society. The United States is not alone in feeling these concerns. Most of the mature industrial economies of the world are apprehensive about the ability to sustain economic growth in the face of world competition. At this time, however, no solid data exist to support the notion that we simply cannot afford to provide Social Security to the baby boomers as they age (Schulz, 1997). In fact, many analysts have concluded that very modest increases in tax rates or using some portion of the surplus now would eliminate any projected deficits in the Social Security retirement and survivors programs prior to 2050, the end-point of official projections (Schulz, 1997). However, these facts have not stopped those who oppose social insurance on ideological grounds from continuing a well-financed campaign to lower the public's confidence in Social Security.

Medicare is in need of substantial reform. Current levels of expenditure are expected to deplete the Medicare Trust Fund by shortly after the year 2000. Yet the issues involved in reforming Medicare are exceedingly complex, and there is wide disparity in the solutions being proposed. Many observers expect that, irrespective of how the system is revised, there will be an erosion in access to and adequacy of health services for a large majority of older Americans.

The responsibility for Medicaid financing rests on individual states and their willingness to appropriate tax dollars for the state's share of Medicaid funding. Most state policymakers believe it will not be possible to sustain the growth in Medicaid funding required to meet the increasing need for long-term care among a growing population of low-income elders. To reduce or at least contain financial commitments to Medicaid, states are looking to home- and community-based solutions, which often shift the cost and the responsibilities to families, regardless of their capacities to provide assistance. As a result, waiting lists have increased for all types of Medicaid-funded long-term care services, including nursing facility placement, assisted living, home care services, and adult day care.

Eroded Confidence in Government

Thus, even though economic growth has been steady, the public remains ambivalent about increasing taxes to meet common societal needs. Part of this unwillingness may be manufactured by legislators and other public policymakers to justify ideologically driven government withdrawals from a wide range of social commitments, including education, housing, transportation, science, and a host of others in addition to programs affecting the older population. For example, a very large majority of the public supports increased taxation to preserve the Social Security retirement program in its present form (Cook & Barrett, 1992), but influential politicians cite the public's unwillingness to pay additional taxes as the rationale for cutbacks or reforms in Social Security. Nevertheless, part of the public's ambivalence about paying more taxes is based on low confidence in elected government officials.

Media coverage of a seemingly endless series of scandals involving alleged misconduct or mismanagement by public officials, the most notable of which was the Watergate affair, has certainly eroded public trust in government. But perhaps a more important factor has been the inability of elected officials to bring a sense of fairness to taxation, interest group politics, and campaign finance. The existing tax system in the United States dramatically favors those who are economically advantaged, and, despite political rhetoric to the contrary, such tax inequality is considerably higher today than in the mid-1960s (Barlett & Steele, 1992). In addition, interest group politics and campaign finance issues have combined to produce apparent favoritism in public expenditures and in the relaxation of regulations designed to protect the public. Yet, policymakers have not been able to reform the rules under which interest groups operate or campaigns are financed. So long as legislators are unwilling to address these issues of fairness, the public can be expected to continue to perceive government as lacking the integrity to seek fair solutions to societal needs. This negative attitude affects the prospects for all collective responses to societal problems, including those of concern both to the field of aging and to the vision and blindness systems.

Howard (1994) noted that public confidence in government's ability to address societal problems also has been eroded by a dramatic increase in the use of detailed regulations instead of the traditional "prudent person" test of commonsense decision-making. By micromanaging social concerns through intricate legislation and implementation rules, government at all levels has focused attention on the letter rather than on the purpose of the rule. The results are often inadvertently comical but at the same time produce a loss of public faith in government capability.

Preoccupation with Deficits

A recent political cartoon depicted Congress as being afflicted with "Deficit Attention Disorder." Certainly the federal debt, which grew most substantially during the Reagan and Bush administrations, is a legitimate cause for concern. But legitimate concerns about the deficit and national debt came to be used in political rhetoric in suspect ways, including as an attack on all government programs, regardless of their relationship to the federal budget. For example, Social Security was attacked as an "entitlement" that was preventing Congress from taming the deficit, even though completely eliminating Social Security would not affect the federal government's operating budget, because Social Security revenues are not available for discretionary spending. The word "entitlement" came to possess a negative connotation, and people, no matter how deserving, who benefitted from federal programs of any kind came to be perceived as freeloaders. This rhetorical climate has had a decidedly negative influence on the field of aging, forcing advocates for programs and services to argue the basic legitimacy of income security and care programs rather than focusing their efforts on finding better and more cost-effective solutions.

Decline of the Middle Class

The size of the vast middle class of the United States has been shrinking for at least two decades. The basic causes rest in the restructuring of the American economy into smaller, more autonomous units in which workers' pay is lower, and benefits such as health care insurance and retirement pensions are more problematic. This, in turn, has resulted in more breadwinners working more hours or holding more than one job just to remain at the same level (Rifkin, 1995). People who are struggling to maintain their basic way of life are often less sympathetic to the needs of the disadvantaged, and since 1980 the growing financially precarious population within the middle class has certainly become less sympathetic to the needs of the older population. Part of their lack of sympathy is based on their fear that, by the time they need retirement income or health care in old age, those programs will have become depleted, which of course is linked with their distrust of government.

Hopelessness

Finally, the sheer size of the baby-boom population cohorts has induced an attitude of hopelessness in many people. If difficulties in providing income security, health care, and long-term care to the nation's elders exist now, how will it be possible to provide for the needs of the much larger baby-boom population? Such simplistic thinking is seductive, but it ignores several important facts. First, the baby boom occurred over a period of 20 years, and only part of the baby-boom population will be in the highest-need age categories at any given time. The baby boom is not like a tidal wave, which advances all at once. Second, real wages historically have increased faster than retirement income, even for indexed pensions, which means that Social Security taxes from a smaller number of workers can potentially be sufficient to provide Social Security benefits to a larger number of retirees. Third, active life expectancy—the proportion of later life that is led in a relatively active and healthy state—is increasing rapidly, which could potentially reduce pressures on health care expenditures. In addition, efforts to promote healthy living by curtailing use of tobacco, adopting healthy diets and regular exercise, and encouraging other preventive health measures appear to pay off, resulting in delayed onset and lower prevalence of chronic illness and disability. These are just a few examples of trends that could soften the impact of the baby-boom population on national resources. They are not intended to minimize the need to plan for the baby-boom population as it ages but simply to suggest that the situation is far from hopeless.

A FUTURE AGENDA FOR THE FIELD OF AGING

Forecasting the future is always risky, but it is possible to suggest a few trends that are likely to be the focus of attention in the field of aging over the next decade:

- ✦ Because of the social, economic, and political climate, the field of aging is likely to be preoccupied over the next decade with protecting gains achieved in the past. A great deal of energy within the field of aging probably will be spent trying to oppose efforts by policymakers to subject Social Security and Medicare to a means test, because most advocates believe that means testing might destroy the currently high public support these programs enjoy.
- ✦ Health care rationing is a way of life now, and the field of aging can be expected to vigorously oppose the categorical denial of access to health or care services based on age.
- ✦ The concept of managed care is predominating in the field in both health and personal care services, but it is still largely unknown how to translate the concept of managed care into effective operations. A great deal of energy probably will go into gathering data that can be used to assess various managed care approaches.
- ✦ Emphasis will increasingly be placed on personal responsibility with regard to such issues as retirement income, housing needs, service needs, and service management. People probably will be expected to support themselves financially to a greater extent,

find their own affordable housing, and figure out where and how to obtain the services they need. This trend may occasionally be accompanied by training to enable individuals to assume these responsibilities effectively, but most people are likely to be left to fend for themselves, which many simply will be unable to do. Such an outcome, in turn, will put increased pressures on local, non-government-funded social service agencies. This trend will be accompanied by a decrease in public dialogue on these issues and a decreased sense of collective public responsibility for negative outcomes that result from the lack of an adequate, integrated service delivery system.

◆ More health and personal care services probably will be provided by a deregulated private sector, which, when tied to individual responsibility for service management, may increase the potential for fraud and abuse. This is not to say that services should not be provided for profit, but when the individuals are responsible for coordinating services for themselves, they have little protection against unscrupulous providers.

◆ An important new direction for the field of aging is a growing emphasis on prevention, intervention, rehabilitation, and compensation for loss in the area of conditions that cause functional disabilities in the older population. There are potentially great opportunities for alliances with the vision and blindness systems in this area.

◆ The focus of advocacy in the field of aging will shift from preoccupation with support at the federal level to an emphasis on the state level.

◆ A critical question for the field of aging is how to recruit, train, and retain the needed personnel to provide high-quality services to an aging population.

◆ Changing needs and resources in the older population mean a continued demand for high-quality research to provide the information needed for decision making. Some of the questions that need to be answered are:

  ◆ How much need exists for programs and services of various kinds?

- ◆ What service models work best? Do some services do more harm than good? What is the most cost-effective way to offer specific services?
- ◆ What values take precedence in making policy decisions about what services to fund and at what level?
- ◆ Does regulation work, or is it necessary to find other ways to control fraud and abuse in the field of aging?

Professionals can make more or less well educated guesses about the answers to these questions, but there is no substitute for objective research as a resource for making important decisions about policy and practice. (See also Chapter 10 on "Directions for Research in Aging and Vision Rehabilitation.")

COMMON GROUND BETWEEN AGING AND THE VISION AND BLINDNESS SYSTEMS

As mentioned earlier, many people who work in the field of aging have little understanding of how issues of vision, visual impairment, low vision, or blindness interact with the issues they define as central. Yet in reality, virtually every aspect of the field of aging is influenced at least to some degree by vision-related issues. For example, some might consider income security in later life to be an issue with little tie to vision. But systems for generating retirement income are based on an assumption that disability is rare prior to age 62, and disability income is usually considerably less than retirement income from the same job. Thus, low vision in early or middle adulthood can drastically affect current income, potential disability income, and future retirement income.

To begin to see the links between vision issues and other issues related to aging, those in the field of aging need to be educated concerning the types of vision-related issues and their age-related prevalence. It is important to know more about:

- ◆ The prevalence of various visual impairments and the risk factors associated with them

- ◆ The interrelationships between visual impairments and age-related forms of disability
- ◆ How visual impairments can be prevented
- ◆ How the processes of aging interact with programs designed to help people compensate for low vision or blindness
- ◆ Assistive technology that can help compensate for visual impairment
- ◆ What service providers and family members need to know to help family members who are coping concurrently with visual impairments and other disabilities

Professionals in the field of aging also need to learn what issues are seen as most important within the vision and blindness systems and how those issues can be articulated with the agenda of the field of aging. Gerontologists need readily understandable resources that pull together the necessary information needed to include vision issues in the context of prevention, intervention, rehabilitation, care, and compensation for an aging population. This book is an important step in that direction.

REFERENCES

Atchley, R. C. (2000). *Social forces and aging* (9th ed.). Belmont, CA: Wadsworth.

Barlett, D. L., & Steele, J. B. (1992). *America: What went wrong?* Kansas City: Andrews and McMeel.

Branch, L. G., Coulam, R. F., & Zimmerman, Y. A. (1995). The PACE evaluation: Initial findings. *The Gerontologist, 35,* 349–359.

Cook, F. L., & Barrett, E. N. (1992). *Support for the American welfare state: The views of Congress and the public.* New York: Columbia University Press.

Horowitz, A. (1994). Vision impairment and functional disability among nursing home residents. *The Gerontologist, 26,* 316–323.

Howard, P. K. (1994). *The death of common sense: How law is suffocating America.* New York: Random House.

Hoyert, D. L., & Seltzer, M. M. (1992). Factors related to the well-being and life activities of family caregivers. *Family Relations, 41,* 74–81.

Kahn, R. A., Liebowitz, H. W., Ganley, S. P., Kini, M. M., Colton, J., Nickerson, R. S., & Dawber, T. R. (1977). Framingham Eye Study I: Outlines and major prevalence and findings. *American Journal of Epidemiology, 11,*17–32.

Kline, D. W., & Scialfa, C. T. (1996). Visual and auditory aging. In J. E. Birren & K. W. Schaie (Eds.), *Handbook of the psychology of aging* (4th ed.). New York: Academic Press, pp. 181–203.

Markides, K. S. (1989). *Aging and health: Perspectives on gender, race, ethnicity and class.* Newbury Park, CA: Sage.

Mehdizadeh, S. A., Kunkel, S. R., & Applebaum, R. A. (1996). *Projections of Ohio's disabled older population.* Oxford, OH: Scripps Gerontology Center.

Neugarten, B. L. (1982). *Age or need? Public policies for older people.* Beverly Hills, CA: Sage.

Newcomer, R. J., Harrington, C., Manton, K. J., & Lynch, M. (1995). A response to representatives from the social HMOs regarding program evaluation. *The Gerontologist, 35,* 292–294.

Pynoos, J., & Parrott, T. (1996). The politics of mixing older persons and younger persons with disabilities in federally assisted housing. *The Gerontologist, 36,* 518–529.

Rifkin, J. (1995). *The end of work: The decline of the global labor force and the dawn of the post-market era.* New York: G. P. Putnam's Sons.

Scala, M. A., & Mayberry, P. S. (1997). *Consumer-directed home services: Issues and models.* Oxford, OH: Scripps Gerontology Center.

Scheiber, F. (1992). Aging and the senses. In J. E. Birren, R. Sloane, & G. D. Cohen (Eds.), *Handbook of mental health and aging* (2nd ed.). New York: Academic Press, pp. 251–306.

Schulz, J. H. (1997). The real crisis of the century: Growing inequality, not stealing from our children. *The Gerontologist, 37,*130–131.

Spore, D. L., & Atchley, R. C. (1990). Ohio mental health center directors' perceptions of programming for older adults. *Journal of Applied Gerontology, 9,* 36–52.

U.S. Bureau of the Census. (1992). *Projections of the U.S. population by age and sex: 1990–2050.* Current Population Reports (Series P-25, No. 1092). Washington, DC: US Government Printing Office.

CHAPTER 2

Aging and Vision Loss: A Conceptual Framework for Policy and Practice

John E. Crews

Last summer, as my family and I made our annual driving trip from Atlanta to visit my parents in north central Indiana, we turned off the freeway to take a local highway through small farm communities. As we drove through the Indiana town of Greensburg, in the hot, humid July weather, we passed—in a few fleeting seconds—an old man and an old woman mowing their lawn in the mid-day heat. The couple were at least in their late 80s, and they were dressed far too warmly for the hot summer day. The old man pushed a small power lawnmower up a small knoll, while his wife pulled a rope fastened to the front of the mower. The image was fleeting but powerful.

This couple struggled to perform this most mundane activity. They contributed their combined energy and ingenuity, working together to do something they both deemed important.

Someone else might have called a lawn service or employed a neighbor's child to do the work, but the particular task is unimportant. It is not known why this couple chose to expend their limited energy on this chore. The image, however, capturing them as it does in their struggle to maintain independence, suggests some important themes about aging. These themes, as applied to the subjects of aging, vision loss, and rehabilitation, might be stated as follows:

- ◆ Vision loss is a profoundly personal experience.
- ◆ Vision loss has implications not only for the individual but also for family members and caregivers.
- ◆ Older people who lose vision want to continue the activities that are important *to them.*
- ◆ The ability to continue a few activities may have great implications for improved or sustained quality of life.

Yet, despite the personal nature of vision loss among older people, it occurs within the context of very broad social and economic circumstances that must be fully understood before effective policy and practice can be formulated:

- ◆ The aging population is growing both in absolute numbers and as a proportion of the general population in the United States and other industrialized countries.
- ◆ As the population ages, more people will develop age-related disabilities that compromise their quality of life.
- ◆ As the nation ages, proportionately fewer working-age people will be available to fund social programs, provide economic security, and assume caregiving responsibilities.
- ◆ At this point in history, political trends preclude the likelihood of increased government funding for additional social service or rehabilitation programs, regardless of the gravity of the need.

Moreover, vision loss among older people occurs in a context in which the rehabilitation and social service organizations that are expected to respond to the needs of people who are blind and visually impaired often do not have the capacity or resources to attend to consumers' needs. Rehabilitation services for older people are based not on need but rather on the resources available in the state and community. Federal funding for rehabilitation services remains seriously inadequate for the great need defined by a growing population, but third-party reimbursement has yet to emerge as a method to pay for rehabilitation services, low vision aids, and adapted equipment.

The evolution of public policies to serve older people experiencing vision loss has been hampered by two major factors. One has to do with policies that equated vision rehabilitation with vocational rehabilitation, in which a job was the desired outcome. Thus, rehabilitation was not associated with older people. The second factor has to do with the great uncertainty regarding the number of older people who experience vision problems.

Each of these circumstances will be discussed in more detail in the sections that follow in order to create a conceptual framework that can inform the discussion of policy and practice in the area of vision and aging.

AGING IN THE UNITED STATES

Fundamental shifts are occurring in the United States as a result of a rapidly aging population. The number of people living into old age is increasing rather dramatically. For example, in 1900 there were 3,084,000 Americans (4 percent of the population) over the age of 65; in the year 2000, that number is expected to be 34,882,000 (13 percent of the population). By the year 2030, an estimated 65,604,000 people (21.8 percent of the population) will be over age 65 (U.S. Senate Special Committee on Aging, 1991). The year 2030 is important because by then all of the baby boomers will have joined the ranks of elders. Because these people are already living, these estimates can be made with a strong level of certainty. Table 1 displays actual and projected increases in the number of people over the age of 65 during the 20th century and the beginning of the 21st, as well as the percentage of the population they represent.

In addition to an increase in numbers, more subtle changes will create policy dilemmas. For example, it is the oldest individuals (those over age 85) who represent the fastest growing population cohort in the United States. Moreover, the mean age of the national population continues to increase because the *proportion* of younger people in the population is shrinking in relation to that of elders. About 2,000 years ago, the average lifespan was about 33 years. In 1900, the average lifespan in the United States was 47 years. In 1,900 years, the lifespan had increased by 16 years. By 1996, the average lifespan had increased

Table 1
Actual and Projected Growth of the Older Population: 1900–2040 (in thousands)

Year	Total Population	Age (Years)								
		65–74		75–84		85+		65+	
		Number	Percent	Number	Percent	Number	Percent	Number	Percent
1900	76,303	2,189	2.9	772	1.0	123	0.2	3,084	4.0
1920	105,711	3,464	3.3	1,259	1.2	210	0.2	4,933	4.7
1940	131,669	6,375	4.8	2,278	1.7	365	0.3	9,019	6.8
1960	179,323	10,997	6.1	4,633	2.6	929	0.5	16,560	9.2
1980	226,546	15,580	6.9	7,729	3.4	2,240	1.0	25,549	11.3
2000	268,266	18,243	6.8	12,017	4.5	4,622	1.7	34,882	13.0
2020	294,364	30,973	10.5	14,443	4.9	6,651	2.3	52,067	17.7
2040	301,807	30,808	10.2	25,050	8.3	12,251	4.1	68,109	22.6

Source: Adapted from *Aging in America: Trends and Projections* (1991). Washington, DC: U.S. Department of Health and Human Services (DHHS Publication No. [FCoA] 91,28001).

to 76 years; thus, in the last century, Americans have gained 27 additional years of life (Brandt & Pope, 1997).

The aging of the American society creates an important and complex frame within which to consider vision loss. It is important to recognize "normal" aging and the changes that normal aging implies (see Chapter 5). Older people represent great variability as a group. A person age 65 who is healthy and financially well off is quite different from a person of the same age who has poor health and modest resources. Moreover, as noted in Chapter 1, the situation of an individual at age 85 or 90 is simply different from that of someone 25 years younger.

Rowe (1985) observes that, as people get older, they become *less* like each other. Diversity among older people results from environmental, biological, genetic, and behavioral-lifestyle risk factors. People who smoke, drink, eat too much, and participate in risky behaviors simply pay a price over time. A group of 5 year olds look pretty much alike; a group of 85 year olds would be quite different. Specific subgroups can be readily identified, including the 5 percent of older people who live in long-term care facilities. Increasingly, both demographers and policymakers understand the great rifts among older people who are defined by gender, health, financial resources, and caregiving needs and responsibilities. For example, women generally do not fare well in old age. They have fewer retirement benefits, they can expect to live many years without a spouse, and they can generally expect to live with more years of disability. Because of the way caregiving responsibilities are distributed in this society, women may spend many years in a caregiving role, only to find that no one is left to care for them when they require support.

The traditional age of retirement at age 65 was selected arbitrarily as a part of the social policies developed in Germany by Bismarck in the 1880s. There was no particular reason for selecting this age, except that few people lived to age 65, and if they lived that long, they could expect only a very short period of retirement. For example, in 1900 only 39 percent of White American males lived to be 65; of those who did, the average life expectancy was 11.9 more years (U.S. Senate Special Committee on Aging, 1991). Although it is often believed that intergenerational family groups were common at that time, with the grandmother living with children and grandchildren and contributing to the life of the family, such arrangements were often short term. Today, by contrast, 75 percent of White men live to be 65, and they can expect to live an additional 16.9 years. For those Americans who are healthy and affluent, the retirement age of 65 today often ushers in a long period of relaxation and productivity.

AGING AND DISABILITY

Despite the increasing possibilities for a long and productive retirement, the public's perception of old age in many respects is a negative stereotype of decline, dependence, and the development of chronic disabling conditions. Therefore, understanding, embracing, and honoring the complexity of age-related disability among older people defines the challenge of establishing sound policy and practice in regard to older persons. Professionals in the field need to be cautious about either overstating or understating the meaning and implication of impairments as they develop in later years.

Age does not *cause* disability, but it does *predict* it. The complexity of disability among older people mirrors the complexity and variability of the aging population. For example, the prevalence of many chronic disabling conditions increases with age (see Table 2). The older a person becomes, the greater the likelihood that he or she will develop chronic age-related impairments (Brummel-Smith, 1990).

Many age-related impairments, however, do not predict a person's inability to function independently, that is, activity limitation. For example, many people who experience impairments such as arthritis and hypertension manage them successfully with appropriate medication and lifestyle changes. Other, less common impairments, such as Parkinson's disease, have the potential to create devastating implications for task performance and independence. In addition, the number of impairments does not necessarily predict overall perception of health or well-being. In fact, focusing on specific impairments may be misleading. Most older people report their health as good or excellent, and they characterize themselves as functioning well (Gilford, 1988).

Table 2
Prevalence of Chronic Conditions, U.S. Civilian
Noninstitutionalized Population, Age 65+, 1991

Chronic Conditions	Prevalence (percentage)		
	Total	65–74	75+
Arthritis	48.4	42.5	57.5
Hypertension	37.2	37.6	36.5
Hearing impairment	32.9	26.6	40.3
Heart disease	29.5	25.6	35.4
Vision disease (cataract, glaucoma)	23.0	17.3	31.6
Vision impairment	7.9	5.6	11.3
Orthopedic impairment	17.7	16.7	19.3
Diabetes	9.9	10.3	9.2
Atherosclerosis	4.2	3.6	5.2
Varicose veins	7.9	9.0	6.2
Cerebrovascular disease	6.3	5.8	7.0
Chronic sinusitis	13.9	15.6	11.3
Emphysema/chronic bronchitis	8.4	8.8	7.8

Source: Reprinted with permission from Jette, A. M. (1995). Disability trends and transitions. In R. H. Binstock & L. K. George (Eds.), *Handbook of Aging and the Social Sciences* (4th ed.). San Diego: Academic Press.

Moreover, most older people utilize compensatory strategies to continue valued activities; some of these strategies are so seamless that they are not noticed. Using an elevator to avoid steps, for example, or driving during daylight hours and avoiding rush-hour traffic can be successful, if unnoticed, adaptations. It is important, therefore, to focus attention on function, perception of well-being, and the ability to continue valued activities (Gignac & Cott, 1998), rather than enumerating diseases or the chronic nature of age-related impairments.

Rates of Disability

A number of recent studies (Crimmins, Saito, & Ingegneri, 1997; Crimmins, Saito, & Reynolds, 1997; Freedman & Martin, 1998; Manton, Corder, & Stallard, 1997), suggest that the rates of disability among older people may be decreasing. Although analyses of data sets from the 1970s and early 1980s suggested that the rates of disability were increasing among older people (Pope & Tarlov, 1991), examination of data sets from the 1980s and early 1990s indicates shifts in the disabling characteristics of older people. Rates may now be decreasing; however, there is little indication that the absolute number of older people with disabilities is likely to decrease in the near term. Nevertheless, given the rapidly increasing older population, declining rates mean that the magnitude of disability among older people may not be as significant in the coming decades as once believed. The implications for family caregiving, Social Security, and health care financing are potentially great.

Manton et al. (1997) examined the National Long-Term Care Survey data from 1982 to 1994 and found that rates of disability declined 0.27 percent a year between 1982 and 1989, and further declined 0.34 percent in each year between 1989 and 1994. Decreases occurred across population cohorts. Manton estimated that in 1982, there were 6.4 million people with chronic disabilities; by 1989, the population had increased to 7.0 million instead of 7.5 million as projected, and by 1994, the number had grown to 7.1 million, rather than 8.3 million persons. Manton estimated that the cost savings in institutional care for 1994 alone was $17.3 billion as a result of these changing rates of disability. These authors suggest that one factor leading to decreasing rates of disability is the effect of better educated cohorts who are more likely to adopt healthy behaviors, seek medical care, and comply with complex medical treatment, thus potentially delaying the onset of disability.

Other scholars who have examined large national data sets have arrived at similar conclusions. Crimmins, Saito, and Reynolds (1997) examined the Longitudinal Study on Aging and found little evidence of sustained decreases in the prevalence of disability, but when examining National Health Interview Survey data, Crimmins, Saito, and Ingegneri (1997), using the broad concept of active life expectancy, found that increasing years of life expectancy were accompanied by additional years free of disability. Similarly, when Freedman and Martin (1998) examined discrete task performance (in seeing, lifting, walking, and getting into or out of a bed or chair), they were able to demonstrate decreasing rates of disability as well.

Disease, Disability, and Life Expectancy

Perhaps a useful way to understand the sequence of events associated with the onset of disability among older people is to employ a framework from a life table model (Manton & Soldo, 1985). In Figure 1, the *morbidity* curve represents years that members of a population cohort are expected to live without chronic disease. The area under the morbidity curve represents years of *healthy life expectancy*. The curve labeled *disability* represents the probability of surviving to a given age without disability, and the total area under the disability curve represents *active life expectancy*. The area between morbidity and disability represents years spent ill but not disabled. The area between disability and mortality represents years spent with a disability. This model suggests that illness and disability are equated once disability occurs, but that is misleading because people can be disabled and healthy. Finally, the mortality curve represents total years in life, and as noted earlier, lifespan increased dramatically since 1990. Historically, these curves have moved increasingly toward the upper right corner of the

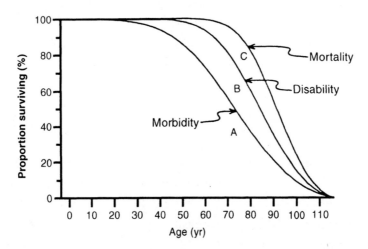

Figure 1
Morbidity, Disability, and Mortality Survival Curves

Source: Manton, K., & Soldo, B. J. (1985). Dynamics of health changes in the oldest old: New perspectives and evidence. *Millbank Memorial Fund Quarterly—Health and Society, 63,* 206–285. Reproduced with permission.

table, becoming increasingly rectangular, as life expectancy, active life expectancy, and healthy life expectancy have increased throughout the 20th century as public health, medical care, and lifestyle changes have influenced the life course of Americans.

Crimmins, Saito, and Ingegneri (1997) explore this concept further in a recent examination of active life expectancy using data from the National Center for Health Statistics National Health Interview Survey data for 1970, 1980, and 1990. Over this 20-year period, they were able to demonstrate increasing life expectancy as well as increasing active life expectancy from cross-sectional data on older people. Table 3 shows estimated total life expectancy, years spent nondisabled, years spent disabled and living in the community, and years spent institutionalized for people at birth, at age 65, and at age 85.

Examining the experience of people at age 65 is instructive. In the 1970s, men gained 1.2 years of life; of that, 1 year was spent living with a disability in the community and an additional 0.1 of a year living in an institution. Of the total 1.2 years of additional life, only 0.2 of a year were free of disability. In the 1970s, women did not fare well. Although women gained 1.6 years of life, nearly all of it, 1.4 years, consisted of living with a disability in an institution. Like men, women gained 0.2 of a year of disability-free years. The 1980s presented a different picture. Men at age 65 gained an additional 0.9 of a year of life, most of which was free of disability, and the period of institutionalization did not increase. Women, in some respects, did better. Although women gained only 0.5 of a year of additional life, all of it was disability-free time, and, in fact, years in an institution declined.

These demographic changes suggest that the survival curve continues to move outward with more years of life. Fries (1980, 1988) suggested that a compression of morbidity may occur as years without a disability move closer to years of survival. Crimmins notes that her data suggest that a compression of morbidity occurred among older age groups in the 1980s.

As more is understood about aging and disability, it is clear that individual experiences are as broad as the human condition will allow. The factors that define aging and disability are so great that stereotypes have unwittingly been created to simplify human experience.

Table 3
Expectation of Life (in Years) Spent in Various States of Health, at Birth, at Age 65, and at Age 85, by Sex: United States 1970, 1980, 1990

Expectation of Life	Men			Change		Women			Change	
	1970	1980	1990	1970–80	1980–90	1970	1980	1990	1970–80	1980–90
At birth										
Total	67.0	70.1	71.8	3.1	1.7	74.6	77.6	78.8	3.0	1.2
Nondisabled	56.5	57.2	58.8	0.7	1.6	62.7	62.8	63.9	0.1	1.1
Disabled and living in the community	10.0	12.2	12.4	2.2	0.2	10.9	13.4	13.4	2.5	0.0
Institutionalized	0.6	0.6	0.7	0.0	0.1	1.1	1.4	1.4	0.3	0.0
At age 65										
Total	13.0	14.2	15.1	1.2	0.9	16.8	18.4	18.9	1.6	0.5
Nondisabled	6.6	6.8	7.4	0.2	0.6	9.1	9.3	9.8	0.2	0.5
Disabled and living in the community	5.8	6.8	7.0	1.0	0.2	6.6	7.6	7.5	1.0	-0.1
Institutionalized	0.5	0.6	0.6	0.1	0.0	1.1	1.5	1.5	0.4	0.0
At age 85										
Total	4.7	5.1	5.2	0.4	0.1	5.6	6.4	6.4	0.8	0.0
Nondisabled	1.4	1.5	1.6	0.1	0.1	1.4	1.7	1.6	0.3	-0.1
Disabled and living in the community	2.7	2.8	2.7	0.1	-0.1	3.0	3.0	3.0	0.0	0.0
Institutionalized	0.6	0.8	0.9	0.2	0.1	1.2	1.7	1.8	0.5	0.1

Source: Reprinted with permission of the Population Council, from Crimmins, E. M. et al., Trends in disability-free life expectancy in the United States, 1970–1990. *Population and Development Review,* Vol. 23, No. 3 (September 1997), 555–572.

Pope and Tarlov (1991) observe, "Public attitudes toward the aging process have fostered an unduly pessimistic view of the late stage of adulthood" (p. 212). They argue that the concept of aging and disability simply needs to be expanded in ways to embrace the complexity of human experience that includes physical functioning as well as quality of life. Pope and Tarlov (1991) assert:

> Successful aging, or aging well, does not imply freedom from disabling conditions. One is aging well when one maintains a satisfying sense of continuity and can fulfill expectations of personal independence and social participation. Despite the physiological and psychological stresses that can accompany advancing age, many older adults have the vitality and resilience to function at a high level. Moreover, frailty and dependence need not preclude a reasonable quality of life. Conversely, a low quality of life can affect the likelihood of developing a disability. Just as among younger groups, the risk of disability among the elderly is associated with poverty, inadequate education, poor housing, and social isolation.
>
> Therefore, effective management of chronic disease requires an approach that comprehensively addresses not only the individual's health condition but also his or her total social situation. Indeed, beneficial outcomes have been shown to be more likely when personal and social variables are taken into account in geriatric rehabilitation programs. (p. 198)

ESTIMATES OF VISION LOSS AMONG OLDER PEOPLE

The same demographic shifts that are influencing the general population in terms of aging and the onset of age-related disabilities define the environment for older people who experience visual loss. By far, most of the people who experience visual impairment are older people who grew up, worked, reared their families, and retired as sighted people. Although there are several estimates regarding the exact number of older people who experience varying degrees of visual impairment, about 3 million older people have vision loss that prevents them from reading newspaper print. This number is likely to grow to about 6 million by the year 2030 (Crews, 1994). Two interrelated factors will lead to that increase. First, most leading causes of vision impairment—macular degeneration, cataract, diabetes, and glaucoma—are more common among older people, especially those at the oldest ages. Second, the population is aging rapidly, and those aged 85 and over are the fastest-growing age group, thus accelerating the number of people who acquire vision problems.

Table 4 presents a 1991 estimate of the number of people who are over the age of 65 and experience severe visual impairment and projections to the year 2020. Note that in the 1960s, the largest number of people experiencing vision loss were in their 60s. By 1970, the largest cohort had shifted to those in their 70s, and by 2000, the largest cohort will be those over the age of 85.

As noted earlier, the inability to obtain an accurate estimate of the number of older people with vision loss has long been a stumbling block in developing public policy for this group. The lack of accurate estimates is further confused by inconsistent clinical, functional, and self-reported definitions of visual impairment.

Although a number of efforts have attempted to estimate the size of the population of elders who experience vision problems, until recently most of the knowledge about this group has emerged from small-scale studies, state registries, or large multipurpose health surveys. The limitations of these studies have confounded attempts to understand the scale and complexity of the problem. Most people concerned with public policy or service delivery simply want to know "how many" blind people live in a particular community or state. But estimates have never been easy to achieve because the legal definition of blindness is a clinical one (based on measuring visual acuity and visual field), and most data sets generally request a self-report from survey participants. Because the questions regarding visual impairment demonstrate considerable variability, the responses demonstrate remarkable variability as well. Some surveys ask questions about specific functional capacity (the ability to read newspaper print or recognize faces); others ask more general questions such as whether the individual has "any trouble seeing." Still others ask respondents to report if they are "blind."

The major studies attempting to project accurate estimates of the number of people experiencing vision loss include the following:

Table 4
Prevalence of Severe Visual Impairment in Persons Aged 65 and Over, United States, 1960–2020

Age Group	1960	1970	1980	1990	2000	2010	2020
65–74	516,859	584,445	732,307	873,307	830,819	954,946	1,402,245
75–84	458,716	605,781	765,151	1,024,551	1,219,482	1,220,274	1,434,114
85+	232,250	337,750	560,000	828,250	1,231,500	1,637,700	1,770,250
Totals	1,207,825	1,567,976	2,057,458	2,726,108	3,281,801	3,812,920	4,606,609

Source: Reprinted from Crews, J. E. (1991). Strategic planning and independent living for elders who are blind. *Journal of Visual Impairment & Blindness, 85* (2), 52–57.

1973	Model Reporting Area (Kirchner & Lowman, 1988)
1973–1975	Framingham Study (Kahn et al., 1977; Felson et al., 1989)
1980	National Society to Prevent Blindness
1971, 1977	National Center for Health Statistics Health Interview Surveys (Kirchner, 1988)
1984	National Center for Health Statistics 1984 Supplement on Aging (Havlik, 1986; Nelson, 1987; Nelson & Dimitrova, 1993; Crews, 1991, 1994)
1985–1988	Baltimore Eye Survey (Sommer et al., 1991; Tielsch et al., 1990; Tielsch et al., 1991a; Tielsch et al., 1991b; Tielsch et al., 1995; Katz & Tielsch, 1996)
1994	Lighthouse National Survey on Vision Loss
1991–1992	Bureau of the Census, Survey of Income and Program Participation (SIPP) (Schmeidler & Halfman, 1998a)
1994	1994 Second Supplement on Aging (SOA II), (NCHS, 1998a; Campbell et al., 1999)
1994	1994 National Health Interview Survey on Disability, Phase I and II (NCHS, 1998b; Schmeidler & Halfman, 1998b)

In recent years, most researchers have relied on data produced by the National Center for Health Statistics Health Interview Surveys (Kirchner, 1988; Kirchner & Lowman, 1988) and the NCHS 1984 Supplement on Aging (Crews, 1991, 1994; Havlik, 1986; Nelson, 1987; Nelson & Dimitrova, 1993). To appreciate this evolving data problem, one must recognize, in part, that many researchers and policymakers simply could not access or manipulate large data files that are so easily analyzed today with PCs and CD-ROMs. The National Center for Health Statistics, for example, conducts the Health Interview Survey annually, and, although the data set is population based and highly detailed, only a few researchers, most notably Kirchner (1988) and her colleagues, have analyzed these data and presented the findings to users.

For individuals concerned about vision loss and aging, the 1984 Supplement of Aging (SOA) (Havlik, 1986) serves as landmark research. This Health Interview Survey (HIS) gathered self-report information from a large sample of elders regarding a variety of near, intermediate, and distance vision activities, and in addition, the study gathered information about a range of other health problems, activity limitations, and participation measures. The large sample was population based, meaning that weights were attached to the sample to allow researchers to make accurate estimates about the national population.

In 1979 Kirchner examined the 1977 National Center for Health Statistics data and estimated that 990,000 older people had severe vision problems; 8 years later, Nelson (1987) analyzed the 1984 SOA study and estimated a total population of 2,028,000 older people who experienced severe visual impairment. Nelson then observed:

> The proportion of elderly identified in 1984 as blind or otherwise severely visually impaired was much higher than the proportion identified in 1977—7.8 percent compared to 4.5 percent, an increase of 74 percent. The absolute number of severely visually impaired people rose even more. In 1977, NCHS estimated 990,000 elderly Americans were severely visually impaired. By contrast, preliminary estimates from the 1984 study was that over *two million* elderly people were unable to read newspaper print, an increase of 106 percent. (p. 332)

Crews (1991), applying 1984 SOA prevalence rates to 1990 census data, estimated the total population of older people with severe visual impairment to be 2,700,000. Two years later, Nelson and Dimitrova (1993) analyzed the 1984 Supplement on Aging and created a state-by-state estimate of severe vision impairment based on 1990 census data. The estimates in their inquiry showed the total number of severely visually impaired elderly persons (65+) to be 2,900,000. This estimate was nearly triple that obtained from the analysis of 1977 data.

Two additional data sets were made available from the National Center for Health Statistics in late 1998. The 1994 National Health Interview Survey on Disability, Phase I and II, was released in July, 1998, and the Second Supplement on Aging, 1994 (SOA II) was released in September, 1998. Although a number of researchers are actively analyzing these data (Schmeidler & Halfman, 1998), very little has been published. A limitation of the Second Supplement on Aging is that it captures data only for people 70 years of age and over, and although this data set will serve as the foundation for a second Longitudinal Study on Aging, it does not provide detailed information regarding people aged 65 to 69. In that respect, the new SOA II creates difficulties in comparing these new cross-sectional data with other data sets. [The 1984 Supplement on Aging became the foundation for the Longitudinal Study on Aging (LSOA), that is, the first longitudinal study on aging. The 1994 Supplement on Aging is the foundation for the Second Longitudinal Study on Aging. The National Center for Health Statistics is conducting this study.]

Preliminary analysis of the SOA II reveals that 3,652,626 people over the age of 70 reported being blind in one eye, being blind in both eyes, or having any other trouble seeing in 1994. These 3.6 million people represent 18.1 percent of the elders 70 years of age and over (Campbell et al., 1999). By contrast, Havlik (1986) reported that 12.8 percent of those *over age 65* (3,365,000) reported similar limitations with seeing in 1984. Without further analysis, it would appear that the absolute number of elders with vision impairment is increasing. However, conflicting information arises from an examination of the Bureau of the Census's Survey of Income and Program Participation (SIPP) by Freedman and Martin (1998) suggesting that the *rates* of visual impairment may be declining. The SIPP asked respondents if they have difficulty seeing words in newspaper; in the 1984 survey, 15.3 percent of the population over the age of 50 reported difficulty seeing words in the newspaper; in the 1993 survey, only 11.6 percent of respondents over age 50 reported difficulty seeing words. Declines occurred in each age cohort they examined.

To further complicate matters, all the studies mentioned make estimates regarding the community-dwelling population, and elders residing in institutional settings are omitted. With few exceptions (Horowitz, 1994; Kirchner, 1988), research studies have not attempted to estimate the number or characteristics of nursing home residents who experience vision problems. Limitations in the research design, including small sample size, lack of clinical data, high rates of dementia, and lack of eye care, make population estimates very difficult to obtain. A recent study, the Baltimore Nursing Home Eye Survey (Tielsch, Javitt, Coleman, Katz, & Sommer, 1995), is a population-based survey with 738 subjects over the age of 40, almost 70 percent of whom completed at least part of an ocular examination. Tielsch and his colleagues found, as one would expect, that age was strongly associated with visual impairment, and that the rate of blindness among those 90 and over was twice that of those in their 60s. They found the rate of "poor vision (visual impairment or blindness)" to be 35.8 percent among nursing home residents. Rates of visual impairment among Black residents was 50 percent higher than among Whites; and rates among women were greater than among men. Tielsch and his colleagues observe:

> As compared with community dwelling persons of the same age and from the same base population, nursing home residents had a dramatically higher prevalence of blindness. Overall, prevalence of blindness for nursing home residents were 15.6 times higher for whites and 13.1 times higher for blacks. (p. 1207)

These researchers also found that cataract, a treatable eye condition, was the leading cause of visual impairment, and uncorrected refractive errors were "an important source of visual impairment."

Users of these data are understandably likely to experience frustration because of the apparent inability of researchers to respond to the fairly simple problem of estimating the population of older people experiencing vision problems. Each study has limitations, especially in terms of creating a definition of a vision problem, as seen earlier. Moreover, this task is complicated by the apparent changes in the rate of disability. Although rates may decline, the absolute number of people who experience vision problems may not decrease because of the rapidly aging composition of the older population. Despite the lack of definitive statistics, it is possible to state that serious vision problems affect between 3 and 3.5 million older people who reside in the community. The numbers of people who experience dementia are roughly equivalent to the estimates of people who experience vision loss (Brookmeyer, Gray, & Kawas, 1998). Regardless of the precise figure, vision loss is clearly a serious business; it therefore demands access to the various social and medical interventions that have the potential to ameliorate its effects. Estimates over the last 20 years, as mentioned previously, have led researchers to report a threefold increase in the number of people experiencing vision problems; public policies have not responded to those increasing numbers.

SECONDARY CONDITIONS

Another aspect of the context in which aging and vision loss exist— one that is generally poorly understood in the field of vision rehabilitation— is the concept of secondary conditions. A secondary condition is defined as "a condition to which a person is more susceptible by virtue of having a primary disabling condition" that can be either a pathology, an impairment, a functional limitation, or an additional disability (Lollar, 1999). In spinal cord injury, for example, typical secondary conditions include contractures, decubitus ulcers, or impacted bowel (Toal, Burt, & Tomlinson, 1991). Prevention of these secondary conditions among people with spinal cord injury is a major concern of health care, public health, patient education, and public policy (Brandt & Pope, 1997; Graitcer & Maynard, 1990).

Secondary conditions among older people who experience vision loss may be less obvious, in large part because the notion lacks conceptual clarity. Often other health conditions are confused with or reported as secondary conditions. Researchers have identified vision loss as a risk factor leading to functional decline and increased mortality among older people dwelling in the community (LaForge, Spector, & Sternberg, 1992) and to increased risk for imbalance (Gerson, Jarjoura, & McCord, 1989), falls (Daubs, 1973), hip fracture (Felson, Anderson, Hannan, Milton, Wilson, & Kiel, 1989), and depression (Horowitz, 1995; Rovner & Ganguli, 1998; Rovner, Zisselman, & Shmuely-Dulitzki, 1996). Williams, Brody, Thomas, Kaplan, and Brown (1998) demonstrated overall declines in quality of life across several measures of psychosocial well being among older people with macular degeneration.

An examination of the 1994 Supplement on Aging (National Center for Health Statistics, 1998a) shows that older visually impaired people (ages 70–74) are two times as likely to have "difficulty walking" as do sighted people. Moreover, they are more than three times as likely to have difficulty getting outside, more than two times as likely to have difficulty getting into and out of a bed or chair, and more than three times as likely to report difficulty preparing meals than people without vision problems. The connection between vision loss and these activity limitations appears fairly straightforward. If one cannot see well, then one may be less likely to get out of the house or prepare a meal. The *consequences* of these activity limitations, however, are not well understood. As shown in Table 5, findings from the 1994 Supplement on Aging also show that the youngest cohort of older people (70–74) with visual impairment are more likely to experience arthritis or rheumatism (63.5 percent versus 52.8 percent for those with no visual impairment), more likely to experience hypertension (54.1 per-

Table 5
Distribution of People Age 70–74 and 85+ Living in the Community, by Selected Characteristics by Age and Visual Impairment, United States, 1994 (percentage)

| | *70–74 Years* | | *85+ Years* | |
Characteristic	*No Visual Impairment*	*Visual Impairment*	*No Visual Impairment*	*Visual Impairment*
Difficulty walking	15.1	35.7	39.2	55.7
Difficulty getting outside	6.2	20.0	25.4	44.5
Difficult getting in and out of a bed or chair	7.2	17.2	17.6	33.3
Difficulty preparing meals	4.0	13.6	17.1	30.7
Arthritis or rheumatism	52.8	63.5	59.4	68.4
Heart disease	18.0	26.4	21.2	32.1
Hypertension	42.3	54.1	41.8	40.2
Get together with friends	76.0	70.1	59.7	57.9
Get together with relatives	77.9	77.0	70.2	73.7
Go out to eat at restaurant	70.9	61.9	45.6	46.9

Source: Based on data from National Center for Health Statistics (1998a). Data File Documentation, National Health Interview Second Supplement on Aging, 1994 (machine readable data file and documentation). Hyattsville, MD: National Center for Health Statistics.

cent versus 42.3 percent for those with no visual impairment), and *much more* likely to experience cardiovascular disease (33.8 percent versus 19.1 percent for those with no visual impairment).

Vision rehabilitation typically addresses mobility and daily living skills. Increased mobility skills can play a much larger role in an individual's well-being than the concept of traveling from place to place might imply. In addition to getting where one wants to go, an individual has the potential to gain the added benefit that regular exercise creates; conditioning may therefore reduce the risk for cardiovascular disease. The relationship between an individual's well-being and general health and the domain of public policy and public health policy becomes a little clearer when one recognizes that a principal reason many older people with visual impairment do not walk is the lack of sidewalks in the neighborhood (Long, Boyette, & Griffin-Shirley, 1996). Similarly, meal preparation skills, when viewed in a larger context, become increasingly important to an individual's long-term well-being. The lack of adequate skills in meal preparation may lead to an individual becoming overweight on one hand or malnourished on the other. In both cases, the consequences are much graver than is typically assumed in the field of vision rehabilitation.

Further examination of the 1994 SOA reveals some encouraging patterns. Although people with vision problems present greater comorbidities and secondary conditions than older people without visual impairments and although there is great disparity in activity limitations, social participation is not markedly different. Valued activities (see Chapter 6; Gignac & Cott, 1998) such as getting together with friends and relatives and going out to eat are not as dramatically different as activity limitations might predict, but this analysis is incomplete. It is not known if friends and relatives come to the older person who is visually impaired, or if people with visual impairments go to friends and relatives. Information is not available about other valued activities, such as going to church. Although this topic requires additional investigation, these findings suggest that older people are able to employ a variety of strategies that allow them to participate in activities that they deem important.

A study by Jette and Branch (1985) supported the findings from the

1994 Supplement on Aging and Havlik's earlier examination of the 1984 Supplement on Aging (1986). In their investigation of longitudinal data from a large, noninstitutionalized population in the Massachusetts Health Care Panel Study, Jette and Branch examined three impairments: hearing, sight, and musculoskeletal condition. Their instrument examined activities of daily living (ADLs) (walking, bathing, transferring, etc.) and instrumental activities of daily living (IADLs) (housekeeping, preparing meals, grocery shopping, etc.). Their study had two striking findings: (1) older people with vision impairments were significantly more likely to have physical disability, whereas those with hearing impairment were not; and (2) impairment (either vision, hearing, or musculoskeletal) did not predict social isolation; rather, those who lived alone were more likely to be socially isolated than those who did not live alone (p. 62).

In a subsequent study of the same data set, Branch, Horowitz, and Carr (1989) concluded:

> [O]lder people with visual decline are no more likely to use formal social services for health services, but are significantly more likely to report pervasive compromised physical function, diminished social function in selected areas, and uniformly lower emotional function compared to those with continued excellent or good vision. (p. 363)

It is therefore seldom that an older person is concerned only about vision loss; rather, vision loss occurs in the context of other health and mental health concerns, as Kane and Kane (1981) aptly observed:

> Hearing and vision defects, also common in old age, combine with social isolation, depression, and loss of social support systems. Physical, psychological, and social deficits are typically interactive so that it is difficult to distinguish what is causative; but it is clear that a spiral of exacerbations occurs. For example, the presenting picture of a mildly confused individual who walks with difficulty, has a hearing loss, is depressed, and lacks social contacts is not easily unraveled to reveal whether the sensory deficits and immobility have caused the confusion and what part the depression and dwindling social contacts play in the situation. This is the prototype of the patient who typically challenges the geriatrician or

gerontologist; whatever measurements are taken should be targeted to the multiple disabling conditions of such patients and the limitation that these impose for independent daily living. (p. 19)

PUBLIC POLICY, AGING, AND VISION REHABILITATION

In addition to a lack of acurate demographic data, factors such as public attitudes, beliefs, and stereotypes about older people generally and older people with vision problems in particular have led to policies and practices that have denied vision rehabilitation services to older people. Geriatric medicine, like vision rehabilitation for elders, has struggled to define its role and at the same time to define its successes. Frengley (1985) observes:

Clearly, there is no pathologic process that accounts for the many facets of diseases in aging. The likelihood of multipathology must be anticipated: the presence of several chronic conditions simultaneously with an exacerbation of one, a new complication, or the addition of a new diagnosis gives geriatric medicine its singular challenge. (p. 134)

Further, he states:

The goals of medical interventions in the elderly are often very different from those of younger patients; the quality of life rather than the quantity usually dominates the elderly patient's own view of how medical care should be managed. (p. 135)

Among the principles often cited in geriatric medicine are:
◆ Importance of small gains
◆ Use of rehabilitation teams
◆ Individualized rehabilitation programs
◆ Social and peer support

Becker and Kaufman (1988) assert, "Negative cultural forces and economic constraints in the delivery of health care obscure the value of rehabilitation in older people" (p. 466). Becker and Kaufman's comment is directed toward the failure of geriatric rehabilitation to be regarded by mainstream medicine, but their remarks are equally valid for people who require vision rehabilitation.

Vision rehabilitation services, and rehabilitation generally, evolved from models designed to respond to the needs of children and working-aged adults. The events following World War I and World War II led to the development of programs to return veterans to productive work (Wainapel, 1991). Likewise, the polio epidemic following World War II was driven by concerns for productivity defined as work. A powerful argument advanced by vocational rehabilitation was the "payback period." In other words, if rehabilitation services were provided to a 30 year old, he or she might have 35 years of work to "pay back" society in terms of paying taxes, producing goods and services, and exiting the welfare system (Berkowitz, 1985).

For elders, at least two factors mitigate against these notions of payback. First, the payback period might be very short and might not be in terms of productivity measured by work. Second, the general view in America has been to define aging in terms of physical, mental, social, and economic *loss.* Again, Becker and Kaufman assert:

> Because negative assumptions about old age play a part in the delivery of rehabilitation services, questions arise as to whether the American health care system provides incentive for younger patients to regain function but not for older patients; the extent to which cultural values about age affect the patients' own decision making; and whether patients' responses to rehabilitate are age-related? (p. 460)

No comprehensive national policy has evolved regarding visual impairment and aging. Services across the country are inconsistent and unpredictable, and are driven by the resources of particular service providers—not by the needs of consumers. A modest federal commitment of approximately $11 million (in 1998) has been provided to the state rehabilitation agencies, thus affording some presence to vision rehabilitation services in each of the states. These programs, ranging in funding from $165,000 to $225,000, are generally inadequate to meet the demand for services, even though they are limited to the people who are legally blind. Private agencies typically serve a limited geographic area, and they generally rely on a variety of funding sources to assemble community services. The Department of Veterans Affairs, although providing superb services, targets veterans who meet various eligibility criteria. Vision rehabilitation services are therefore driven not by the need but by the vagaries of community resources. Efforts have been directed to making vision rehabilitation services third-party reimbursable through insurance providers, but these initiatives have been only marginally successful. (See Chapter 8 for a detailed discussion of this issue.)

The quality, comprehensiveness, and degree of vision rehabilitation services may vary dramatically from community to community. Services may very well range from absolutely no services to an information and referral pamphlet to a comprehensive rehabilitation program involving rehabilitation teachers, orientation and mobility (O&M) instructors, low vision specialists, and psychosocial services. This inconsistency is tolerated, although the reasons are unclear. By contrast, an individual who experienced a stroke, for example, could expect fairly consistent and predictable rehabilitation protocols almost anywhere in the country. Although the quality of services is variable, nowhere in the country would a person coping with the effects of a stroke be sent home with only a pamphlet.

As noted earlier, vision loss has been regarded as a normal part of aging, the course of which cannot be altered. In addition, until recently, the numbers of older people experiencing vision problems have been greatly underestimated, thus diminishing the perceived magnitude of the problem. Moreover, vision rehabilitation has essentially evolved from different traditions than medical rehabilitation. Rehabilitation teaching evolved from a charity model designed to teach needy blind individuals to read the Bible and perform routine tasks. Modern vision rehabilitation focused on vocational outcomes, first with returning veterans and later with the civilian population. Services for children initially focused upon state schools for blind people and then on community response in public schools. Each of these service models assumed a beginning, middle, and end to the rehabilitation process. The end point was acquiring a job. Vision rehabilitation for older people often does not have an identifiable end point.

The aging network has largely overlooked the needs of older people with vision loss. The evolution of aging policy has focused upon the very large domains of health care, financial supports, nutrition, and community support services. The needs assessments used to define the priorities for Area Agencies on Aging rarely uncover the particular needs of older people experiencing vision loss; consequently, the concerns of older people with vision problems have not surfaced successfully as a competing issue. The gerontological literature has paid much attention to disability, the course of disability, caregiving responsibilities, and the development of scales to measure ADLs and IADLs. Although vision problems are noted as an issue, it is relatively seldom that they are directly addressed.

The result of this environment is that vision rehabilitation for older adults has not surfaced on the public policy agenda. It has largely been an orphan concern—not owned by either the aging or the medical community and, until recently, occupying a low priority among state and local blind rehabilitation organizations.

THE FUTURE OF SERVICES TO OLDER PEOPLE EXPERIENCING VISION LOSS

As the population of older people experiencing visual impairment continues to increase in a fairly dramatic fashion, the complexity of circumstances faced by older people also will grow. Visually impaired elders enter older cohorts and experience increasingly complex health conditions that place additional challenges on informal support systems. This overwhelming complexity will tax the skill of the medical, aging, and rehabilitation communities to tease out strategies to preserve and increase independence.

In looking toward the future of services to older people who are visually impaired, particular attention is needed in three major areas:

1. The individual and those who care for and about that person

2. Public policy to enhance, integrate, and expand services
3. Research to inform services and decision making.

Consumers and Services

By and large, we have a good understanding of the discrete skills that increase the functional independence of older people with vision loss. Rehabilitation teaching, O&M instruction, and low vision services are fairly well established disciplines, and most seasoned professionals in these areas can successfully adapt instructional strategies to better serve older people. Consumers of these services, however, are likely to become increasingly demanding, especially as baby boomers enter their ranks. The demand for quality and timely services may increase. Likewise, consumers are likely to object to the haphazard, fragmented, and poorly funded service system that is currently in place. Consumer empowerment will increasingly reshape the structure of services to older people.

Moreover, to ensure that these services are properly targeted to the needs of older consumers, the *outcome* of vision rehabilitation must be measured in at least two domains: a *functional domain* that demonstrates increased capacity to perform skills and a *quality of life* domain that integrates consumer participation, empowerment, and well being. We are developing tools that create better measures of functional outcome (Crews & Long, 1997), but we have done little to measure increased quality of life. Pope and Tarlov (1991) assert, "Even when functional capacity cannot be restored, it is indeed possible to improve well being and to facilitate personal autonomy by addressing factors in an individual's social situation."

In addition, genuine concern must emerge to respond to the particular needs of people in caregiving and informal support roles. The demands faced by family members are just as serious as the circumstances of families coping with other disabilities. Support systems and services must be developed to respond to the specific concerns of family members, especially spouses and adult children. Although there is a limited literature on aging, vision loss, and caregiving, our current knowledge indicates the imperative of addressing family concerns (see Chapter 6).

Public Policy

The national policy dialogue regarding services for older people must shift to give adequate attention to the seriousness of the problem presented by more than 3 million older people with severe vision impairment. Additional funding for Title VII, Chapter 2 of the Rehabilitation Act (the authorization of federal funding for state vocational rehabilitation agencies to provide training in independent living skills to older individuals who are blind or severely visually impaired) would allow individual states to increase their attention to rehabilitation activities and build on the capacity, structure, and knowledge of those service providers. Moreover, third-party payment through insurance carriers for vision rehabilitation services (rehabilitation teaching, O&M, low vision, and psychosocial services) must be on a par with that for every other major disabling condition in the United States. Stable funding and expanded funding streams would drive the market of rehabilitation providers to respond to the needs of people who require services.

Research

Finally, we simply must increase the knowledge that informs decision-making and practice. The research in aging and vision loss is scant indeed, and, compared to other disabilities or other groups of people experiencing vision loss, little empirical research exists to guide our actions. Often, as revealed in Chapter 9 and other chapters of this volume, it becomes necessary to glean much of the information about broad psychological and social issues from the general body of aging literature. But, as Silverstone argues in Chapter 6 on family caregiving, the needs of older people with vision loss may not be readily comparable to those of older people with other impairments. It is possible to guess and to speculate, but little is known with certainty.

In addition, the disciplines of low vision, O&M, and rehabilitation teaching are increasing their capacity to track and evaluate the effectiveness of their interventions. Yet, although it is possible to intuitively understand the capacity of O&M and rehabilitation teaching to improve function, and anecdotal information reinforces that belief, there is no array of valid and reliable instruments to track the effectiveness of these interventions, either at the time of delivery or longitudinally over the lifespan. These are critical issues. If vision rehabilitation makes a difference in function and quality of life, standard, valid, and reliable measures are needed to assess outcome, to argue for third-party reimbursement, and advocate for increased federal funding. Low vision rehabilitation perhaps has the best standards for measurement, but increased function and acuity must begin to be tied to increased quality of life. In addition, the technologies that have the potential to assist older people need to be explored with greater rigor. Moreover, assistive technology and disability continue to converge to compensate for functional loss, and as the technology and the user continue to evolve, greater attention should be given to identifying technological solutions among older people. Research on aging needs to attend to issues surrounding vision loss. Clearly, vision loss occurs in the context of aging, and aging and disability, and vision loss needs to be regularly included as a variable in research on aging to better understand the circumstances of older people.

REFERENCES

Becker, G., & Kaufman, S. (1988). Old age, rehabilitation, and research: A review of the issues. *The Gerontologist, 28,* 459–468.

Berkowitz, E. (1985). The cost benefit tradition in vocational rehabilitation. In M. Berkowitz (Ed.), *Analysis of costs and benefits in rehabilitation, final report* (pp. 20–54). Department of Education Contract No. 300-84-0259. New Brunswick, NJ: Rutgers University.

Branch, L. G., Horowitz, A., & Carr, C. (1989). The implications for everyday life of incident self-reported visual decline among people over age 65 living in the community. *The Gerontologist, 29,* 359–365.

Brandt, E. N., & Pope, A. M. (1997). *Enabling America: Assessing the role of rehabilitation science and engineering.* Washington, DC: National Academy Press.

Brookmeyer, R., Gray, S., & Kawas, C. (1998). Projections of Alzheimer's disease in the United States and the public health impact of delaying disease onset. *American Journal of Public Health, 88,* 1337–1341.

Brummel-Smith, K. (1990). Introduction. In B. Kemp, K. Brummel-Smith, & J. W. Ramsdell (Eds.), *Geriatric rehabilitation.* Boston: Little, Brown.

Campbell, V., Crews, J. E., Moriarty, D., Zack, M., & Blackman, D. (1999). Surveillance for sensory impairment, activity limitation, and health-related quality of life for older adults. In L. Kamimoto (Ed.), *Surveillance for selected public health indicators affecting older adults—United States. Morbidity and Mortality Weekly Report Surveillance Summary, 48/SS-8,* 135–150.

Crews, J. E. (1991). Strategic planning and independent living for elders who are blind. *Journal of Visual Impairment and Blindness, 85* (2), 52–57.

Crews, J. E. (1994). The demographic, social, and conceptual contexts of aging and vision loss. *Journal of the American Optometric Association, 65* (1), 63–68.

Crews, J. E., & Long, R. G. (1997). Conceptual and methodological issues in rehabilitation outcomes for adults who are visually impaired. *Journal of Visual Impairment and Blindness, 91* (2), 117–130.

Crimmins, E. M., Saito, Y., & Ingegneri, D. (1997). Trends in disability-free life expectancy in the United States, 1970–1990. *Population and Development Review, 23,* 555–572.

Crimmins, E. M., Saito, Y., & Reynolds, S. L. (1997). Further evidence in recent trends in the prevalence and incidence of disability among older Americans from two sources: the LSOA and NHIS. *Journal of Gerontology: Social Sciences, 52* (2), S59-S71.

Daubs, J. G. (1973). Visual factors in the epidemiology of falls by the elderly. *Journal of the American Optometric Association, 44,* 733–736.

Felson, D. T., Anderson, J. J., Hannan, M. T., Milton, R. C., Wilson, P. W. F., & Kiel, D. P. (1989). Impaired vision and hip fracture: The Framingham Study. *Journal of the American Geriatrics Society, 37,* 495–500.

Freedman, V. A., & Martin, L. G. (1998). Understanding trends in functional limitations among older Americans. *American Journal of Public Health, 88,* 1457–1462.

Frengley, J. D. (1985). The special knowledge of geriatric medicine. *Rehabilitation Literature, 45* (4–5), 133–137.

Fries, J. F. (1980). Aging, natural death, and the compression of morbidity. *New England Journal of Medicine, 303,* 130–135.

Fries, J. F. (1988). Aging, illness, and health policy: Implications of the compression of morbidity. *Perspectives in Biology and Medicine, 31,* 407–428.

Gerson, L. W., Jarjoura. D., & McCord, G. (1989). Risk of imbalance in elderly people with impaired hearing and vision. *Age and Aging, 18,* 31–34.

Gignac, M. A. M., & Cott, C. (1998). A conceptual model of independence and dependence for adults with chronic physical illness and disability. *Social Science in Medicine, 47,* 739–753.

Gilford, D. M. (Ed.). (1988). *The aging population in the twenty-first century: Statistics for health policy.* Washington, DC: National Academy Press.

Graitcer, P. L., & Maynard, F. M. (1990). *Proceedings: First Colloquium on Preventing Secondary Disabilities Among People with Spinal Cord Injuries.* Atlanta, GA: Centers for Disease Control.

Havlik, R. J. (1986). *Aging in the eighties, impaired senses for sound and light in persons age 65 and over: Preliminary data from the Supplement on Aging to the National Health Interview Survey: United States. January–June, 1984.* Advance Data No. 25 (September 19, 1986).

Horowitz, A. (1994). Vision impairment and functional disability among nursing home residents. *The Gerontologist, 34,* 316–323.

Horowitz, A. (1995). Aging, vision loss, and depression: A review of the research. *Aging and Vision News,* 7(1), 1, 6–7.

Jette, A. M. (1996). Disability trends and transitions. In R. H. Binstock & L. K. George (Eds.), *Handbook of Aging and the Social Sciences* (4th ed.). San Diego: Academic Press.

Jette, A. M., & Branch, L. G. (1985). Impairment and disability in the aged. *Journal of Chronic Disability, 38,* 59–65.

Kahn, H. A., Leibowitz, H. M., Ganley, J. P., Kini, M. M., Colton, T., Nickerson, R. S., & Dawber, T. R. (1977). The Framingham Eye Study. *American Journal of Epidemiology, 106* (1), 17–32.

Kane, R. A., & Kane, R. L. (1981). *Assessing the elderly: A practical guide to measurement.* New York: Free Press.

Katz, J., & Tielsch, J. M. (1996). Visual function and visual acuity in an urban adult population. *Journal of Visual Impairment & Blindness, 90,* 367–377.

Kirchner, C. (1988). *Data on blindness and visual impairment in the U.S.: A resource manual on social demographic characteristics, education, employment and income, and service delivery.* (2nd ed.) New York: American Foundation for the Blind.

Kirchner, C. & Lowman, C. (1988). Sources of variation in the estimated prevalence of visual loss. In C. Kirchner (Ed.), *Data on blindness and visual impairment in the U.S.: A resource manual on social, demographic characteristics, education, employment and income, and service delivery* (2nd ed.). New York: American Foundation for the Blind.

Kosorok, M. R., Omenn, G. S., Diehr, P., Koepsell, T. D., & Patrick, D. L. (1992). Restricted activity days among older adults. *American Journal of Public Health, 82,* 1263–1267.

LaForge, R. G., Spector, W. D., & Sternberg, J. (1992). The relationship of vision and hearing impairment in one-year mortality and functional decline. *Journal of Aging and Health, 4* (1), 126–148.

Lighthouse national survey on vision loss: The experience, attitudes and knowledge of middle-aged and older Americans. 1995. New York: The Lighthouse Inc.

Lollar, D. (1999). Clinical dimensions of secondary conditions. In R. J. Simeonsson & L. N. McDevitt (Eds.). *Issues in disability and health: The role of secondary conditions and quality of life.* Chapel Hill, NC: The University of North Carolina, Frank Porter Graham Child Development Center.

Long, R. G., Boyette, L. W., & Griffin-Shirley, N. (1996). Older persons and community travel: The effect of visual impairment. *Journal of Visual Impairment & Blindness, 90,* 302–313.

Manton, K. G. (1989). Epidemiological, demographic, and social correlates of disability among the elderly. *The Milbank Quarterly, 67,* Supplement 2, Pt. 1, 13–58.

Manton, K. G., Corder, L., & Stallard, E. (1997). Chronic disability trends in elderly United States populations: 1982–1994. *Proceedings of the National Academy of Sciences, USA, 94,* 2593–2598.

Manton, K., & Soldo, B. J. (1985). Dynamics of health changes in the oldest old: New perspectives and evidence. *Milbank Memorial Fund Quarterly— Health and Society, 63,* 206–285.

Manton, K. G., Stallard, E., & Corder, L. S. (1998). The dynamics of dimensions of age-related disability 1982–1994 in the U.S. elderly population. *Journal of Gerontology: Biological Sciences, 53A* (1), B59-B70.

National Center for Health Statistics (1998a). Data File Documentation, National Health Interview Second Supplement on Aging, 1994 (Machine readable file and documentation). Hyattsville, MD: National Center for Health Statistics.

National Center for Health Statistics (1998b). *1994 National Health Interview Survey on Disability, Phase I and II* (Series 10, No. 8A). Hyattsville, MD: Centers for Disease Control and Prevention.

Nelson, K. A. (1987). Statistical Brief #35: Visual impairment among elderly Americans: Statistics in transition. *Journal of Visual Impairment & Blindness, 80,* 331–334.

Nelson, K. A., & Dimitrova, E. (1993). Statistical Brief #36: Severe visual impairments in the United States and in each state, 1990. *Journal of Visual Impairment & Blindness, 87,* 80–85.

Pope, A. M., & Tarlov, A. R. (1991). *Disability in America: Toward a national agenda for prevention.* Washington, DC: National Academy Press.

Rovner, B. W., & Ganguli, M. (1998). Depression and disability associated with impaired vision: The MoVIES Project. *Journal of the American Geriatrics Society, 46,* 617–619.

Rovner, B. W., Zisselman, P. M., & Shmuely-Dulitzki, Y. (1996). Depression and disability in older people with impaired vision: A follow-up study. *Journal of the American Geriatrics Society, 44,* 181–184.

Rowe, J. W. (1985). Health care of the elderly. *New England Journal of Medicine,* 827–835.

Schmeidler, E., & Halfman, D. (1998a). Distribution of people with visual impairment by community type, prevalence of disability, and growth of the older population. *Journal of Visual Impairment & Blindness, 92,* 380.

Schmeidler, E., & Halfman, D. (1998b). Race and ethnicity of persons with visual impairment; education of children with disabilities; and living arrangements of older Americans. *Journal of Visual Impairment & Blindness, 92* 539–540.

Sommer, A., Tielsch J. M., Katz, J., Quigley, H. A., Gottch, J. D., Javitt, J., & Singh, K. (1991). Racial differences in the cause specific prevalence of blindness in East Baltimore. *New England Journal of Medicine, 325,* 1412–1417.

Tielsch, J. M., Javitt, J. C., Coleman, A., Katz, J., & Sommer, A. (1995). The prevalence of blindness and visual impairment among nursing home residents in Baltimore. *New England Journal of Medicine, 332,* 1205–1209.

Tielsch, J. M., Sommer, A., Witt, K., Katz, J., & Royall, R. M. (1990). Blindness and visual impairment in an American urban population: The Baltimore eye study. *Archives of Ophthalmology, 108,* 286–290.

Tielsch, J. M., Sommer, A., Katz, J., Royall, R. M., Quigley, H. A., & Javitt, J. C. (1991a) Racial variations in the prevalence of open-angle glaucoma: The Baltimore eye survey. *Journal of the American Medical Association, 266,* 369–374.

Tielsch, J. M., Sommer, A., Katz, J., Quigley, H. A., & Ezrine, S. (1991b). Socieconomic status and visual impairment among urban Americans. *Archives of Ophthalmology, 109,* 637–641.

Toal, S. B., Burt, R. L., & Tomlinson, E. C. (1991). *National Conference on the Prevention of Primary and Secondary Disabilities: Proceedings.* Washington, DC: U. S. Department of Health and Human Services, Centers for Disease Control and Prevention.

U. S. Senate Special Committee on Aging, American Association of Retired Persons, Federal Council on the Aging, and U.S. Administration on Aging. (1991). *Aging America: Trends and projections.*

Vision problems in the U.S. (1980). New York: National Society to Prevent Blindness.

Wainapel, S. F. (1991). A tale of two cultures: Cross-disability perspectives in the care of older adults with combined visual and medical disabilities. In N. Weber (Ed.), *Vision and aging: Issues in social work practice.* New York: Haworth.

Williams. R. A., Brody, B. L., Thomas, R. G., Kaplan, R. M., & Brown, S. I. (1998). The psychosocial impact of macular degeneration. *Archives of Ophthalmology, 116,* 514–520.

CHAPTER 3

The Knowledge Base for Collaboration Between the Fields of Aging and Vision Loss

Alberta L. Orr

The growing number of older Americans experiencing age-related visual impairment requires immediate attention not only from vision professionals, but also from professionals in the aging network, home care providers, staff in long-term care facilities, and allied health professionals. As the older population swells in size, it is also becoming increasingly diverse in age (spanning four decades), ethnicity, service needs, and interests. Professionals across many disciplines need to understand the social impact and functional implications of vision loss for the older person and become familiar with the vision rehabilitation services available to ameliorate those problems.

Older people who are blind or visually impaired typically need services from both the aging and vision rehabilitation service delivery systems; therefore, this population should be viewed as simultaneous consumers of both systems. The most efficient and effective way to serve this group is through a reciprocal, shared, and collaborative partnership in planning and delivering services. Based on this premise, a knowledge base in aging and age-related vision loss is essential for service providers to plan for and serve these older consumers in a way that responds to their particular needs.

Vision loss has become a significant enough problem that we cannot afford to wait until professionals are on the job to educate them about age-related vision loss. People preparing to work with older people in general need to know as much basic information about vision loss and its functional implications as they do about Alzheimer's disease, stroke, hypertension, and heart disease. This is true for students preparing to work specifically with older people, as well as all those entering professional fields where older people are inevitably part of their caseload.

Several key points summarize the significance of age-related vision loss as an important gerontological issue:

1. The population of older people experiencing age-related vision loss is increasing dramatically as the population of older Americans is growing exponentially.

2. Although vision loss is not life threatening like many age-related health conditions receiving the greatest public attention, vision loss does have a profound impact on the quality of life and independent living for older persons, on family members, and on the family unit as a whole.

3. Vision-related rehabilitation services, including low vision services, are often available and can ameliorate the impact of vision loss, but many people—professionals, consumers, and the general public—are unaware that these services exist, who is eligible for the services, and how to obtain them.

4. Older people experiencing vision loss do not inevitably have to become dependent, isolated, helpless, or hopeless. They can learn adaptive techniques and how to use adaptive devices, both optical and nonoptical, to continue to live full and productive lives if they and their family members know how to gain access to vision-related rehabilitation services.

5. Placement in long-term-care facilities is not the answer to what can be the egregious effects of vision loss. Vision-related rehabilitation services in combination with home- and community-based long-term services, when needed, can enable

older people with severe vision problems to continue to live in their own homes and familiar communities and can provide family members with the support they need to continue to assist the older person while minimizing the burden. Lack of availability of family support continues to be the leading factor contributing to nursing home placement, regardless of physical or health condition.

6. Professionals within the vision rehabilitation field need to continue to keep pace with the growing and increasingly diverse population of older persons. Increasing numbers of vision rehabilitation professionals—rehabilitation teachers, orientation and mobility specialists, vision rehabilitation therapists, and low vision therapists—are needed to meet the growing demand for services. These professionals must acquire a knowledge base in gerontology and the implications of age-related eye conditions. More funds are needed for professional preparation programs in these areas.

7. Professionals in the aging and vision fields need to plan now for current and future cohorts of older people with age-related vision loss because the next generation of older persons will have greater expectations of vision rehabilitation.

8. Funding in this country for vision-related rehabilitation services for the older population through the Rehabilitation Act is minuscule in comparison to the need of the population. Third-party reimbursement through the health care system is not available in most cases, and the Older Americans Act rarely provides funding for vision rehabilitation. More targeted public funding and a broader funding base are needed, and therefore, continued advocacy efforts are required.

The purpose of this book is to promote collaboration between the aging and vision fields, and a common knowledge base is the best platform on which to build collaborative partnerships.

This chapter describes the core content areas that comprise the necessary knowledge base for professionals working in the aging and health-related fields, the pressing issues confronting the vision rehabilitation field as it prepares for the new millennium, and how professionals in the aging network and the vision field can collaborate to improve the lives of older people who are blind or visually impaired.

CORE KNOWLEDGE BASE IN AGING AND VISION

Given the growing need among older people for vision-related services (see Chapter 2), it is crucial that professionals in all disciplines who work with older people be aware of common eye conditions among older people, their warning signs and effect on functioning, the impact of vision loss on the individual and on family members, and the nature of vision-related and other services that are available. Moreover, such information needs to be available wherever people are providing services to older people. Yet university gerontological curricula traditionally have not covered age-related vision loss (Griffin-Shirley & Orr, 1993).

To remedy this situation and promote effective, collaborative service delivery by an informed network of professionals, a curriculum designed for both university gerontology programs and in-service training was recently compiled by the author (Orr, 1998a,b). The present chapter seeks to provide readers with a summary of basic knowledge about aging and vision loss and a description of critical issues in the field. Other chapters in this volume present more in-depth treatment of specific areas in the field and offer diverse perspectives to provide professionals with a complete picture of the complex challenges our society now faces.

In brief, the core knowledge base needed by professionals outside the vision field includes the following content areas:

1. Demographics of aging-related vision loss
2. Age-related eye conditions and their functional implications
3. Psychosocial aspects of vision loss of the older person and family members
4. Vision-related rehabilitation services and their impact on successful aging

5. Ways to improve access to vision rehabilitation and support services

Demographics of Age-Related Vision Loss

The prevalence of older people experiencing age-related vision loss has increased dramatically since the 1970s. Unless our current projections are altered dramatically by the success of eye research, the number of older persons experiencing age-related vision loss will double by the year 2030.

Most older people with visual impairments have *low vision*, a degree of vision loss significant enough to interfere with the individual's ability to carry out routine tasks independently. Low vision means the older person has some remaining vision and can learn to make the best use of that vision through a low vision assessment, vision rehabilitation, and instruction in the use of adaptive optical devices (Orr, 1998a). In the 85-and-older age cohort, perhaps as many as one older person in three experiences age-related vision loss (Schmeidler & Halfmann, 1997). Within nursing homes, at least 30 percent of the residents are visually impaired (Schmeidler & Halfmann, 1998). The majority of older persons with vision loss are not totally blind.

Blindness and severe visual impairment have been classified as low-incidence disabilities among children with visual impairments in comparison to children with other disabling conditions. It once was accurate to say that the largest portion of the population who were blind were children. However, now that individuals age 55 and over constitute the largest portion of those who are blind or visually impaired, this classification of "low incidence" no longer applies. The demographics of aging and vision loss within the United States and the phenomenon of "global aging" are gradually reshaping both public policy and service delivery for older people. Those aged 65 and older, numbering 34.1 million in 1998, will reach 70 million by 2030 (Administration on Aging, 1998). Therefore, it is impossible to overlook the growing number of older persons experiencing vision loss. This population requires the attention of major decision makers—

policymakers, funders, service planners, and providers—and an increased awareness among the general public.

Since the 1970s, when the steady growth in the aging population became most apparent, projections have been made about the number of older people who would be visually impaired by the year 2000. It is noteworthy that in each decade the actual figures have exceeded the predictions made for the future. The unprecedented growth and the diversity of the elderly population require prioritization for services, as well as creativity and comprehensiveness on the part of service providers, planners, and administrators.

Members of several ethnic minority groups, particularly, African-American, Hispanic and Latino, and Native American elders, experience higher rates of age-related vision loss than the overall population. For example, the incidence of glaucoma is considerably higher among African-Americans than among Caucasians. African-Americans are five times more likely to experience glaucoma, and the rate of blindness resulting from glaucoma in this group is roughly six times that of the general population (National Advisory Eye Council, 1993). Individuals who are Hispanic, African-American, and Native American are more likely to develop diabetes and its associated diabetic retinopathy. Individuals with diabetes are at a higher risk for developing glaucoma. These two eye conditions, diabetic retinopathy and glaucoma, among the four leading eye conditions associated with the aging process, create the greatest threats for total vision loss. Therefore, it is critical that older people representing these ethnic groups have yearly dilated eye examinations.

The projected growth in these populations, particularly in the elderly Hispanic population, will contribute to the increase in age-related vision loss among older persons. The U.S. Bureau of the Census projects that by 2025, a quarter of the nation's older population will be non-Caucasian (Administraton on Aging, 1998). The fastest growth in the minority older population will occur among those age 85 and older. This projected growth will have profound implications for the health and long-term care systems and for the vision field because the population will be more diverse and complex. Calls for bilingual and bicultural outreach strategies and service delivery will be increasingly necessary to ensure that these older people have equal access to essential rehabilitation services.

Information about several other demographic characteristics (Administration on Aging, 1998) is important to consider in order to plan effectively for the next decades:

- *Life expectancy:* While life expectancy is steadily increasing for both men and women, greater life expectancy associated with women means that age-related vision loss among the 75 and older and 85 and older age groups is primarily a women's issue. Women with age-related vision loss are more likely than men to be living alone with less in-home support available to them.
- *Preventive health care:* Lack of access to preventive health care can be a significant correlate to severe vision problems from glaucoma and diabetic retinopathy, which, if diagnosed early, can be treated, and need not result in total blindness. Older people in the low-income categories living in low-income communities frequently have less access to preventive care. This is also often the case for older people of ethnic minority groups.
- *Income and geography:* Low-income populations in both urban and rural communities frequently have less access to health care in general and vision care more specifically. In remote rural communities older people often have to travel great distances to a low vision clinic, and the fact that the clinic is not in their community may mean it will take them longer to learn that such a service is available.

All these factors serve to reinforce the importance of outreach to these groups as an essential foundation creating access to services.

Implications of Demographic Trends

The growing number of older people experiencing vision loss suggests that service providers are likely to see these older individuals more often. Service providers need to learn to recognize the signs of possible vision loss. The growth in this population has serious implications for the range of home- and community-based long-term services available to older persons with disabilities. Older individuals with impaired vision and their families frequently turn to an agency serving the elderly for advice and resources related to vision. Service providers in the aging network need to be able to respond to these inquiries.

Therefore, an emphasis on strategic outreach is needed for two purposes. One is to publicize the availability of vision rehabilitation services within the community for timely referrals from multiple sources—physicians, allied health professions, home care providers, the aging network, and others. The second purpose is to identify and reach those hidden and hard-to-reach special populations, particularly the growing numbers of older people from ethnic minority groups and those in rural areas who have less access to services because of language, cultural, or geographic barriers.

Eye Conditions, Functional Implications, and Treatment Modalities

It is important for service providers to be familiar with the most common eye conditions affecting older people as well as the impact of each eye condition in terms of the person's ability to do routine tasks. (See Chapter 4 for additional details about eye diseases as well as a diagram of the eye and description of its major structures.)

The four eye conditions commonly associated with aging are macular degeneration, glaucoma, diabetic retinopathy, and cataracts. Another frequent cause of vision loss among older people is stroke.

Age-Related Macular Degeneration

Age-related macular degeneration (ARMD) is the most common eye disease among older persons and is the leading cause of visual impairment among older persons. ARMD occurs most frequently among Caucasians. It is a degenerative condition of the macula, which is the area of the retina responsible for central vision, acute vision, and much of color vision. The macula is a small area in the middle of the retina which is the thin tissue lining the back of the eye. The millions of cells of the macula are sensitive to light. The macula makes vision possible from the center part of the eye. ARMD reduces sharp vision needed to see objects clearly and to perform common tasks such as driving and reading. Older people with macular degeneration report having difficulty seeing things that are straight ahead because of the central field loss. For this reason, older people will have difficulty recognizing faces. Peripheral vision remains good and generally intact. Older persons do not become totally blind from macular degeneration. Low vision devices prescribed by a low vision specialist frequently can enable the individual with macular degeneration to read and do other close work.

Glaucoma

Glaucoma is characterized by increased intraocular pressure, which can cause damage or atrophy of the optic nerve and loss of peripheral vision. Intraocular pressure can be measured by tonometry, the eye examination equipment used to measure the fluid pressure within the eye. Pressure within the eye above a reading of 22 is an indication of possible glaucoma. A pressure check should be a routine part of a comprehensive eye examination for adults age 35 years and over.

There are two types of glaucoma associated with aging: *open-angle* and *closed-angle glaucoma.* Open-angle glaucoma is the type most frequently found in the United States and is detected in its early stages during a routine eye examination. It occurs when the eye's drainage canals gradually become clogged. Closed-angle glaucoma (also called acute glaucoma) typically has a sudden onset and is characterized by pain in the eye and blurred vision. Glaucoma is especially dangerous because open-angle glaucoma progresses without pain or obvious symptoms. This is why it is referred to as the "sneak thief of sight." An eye care professional can diagnose glaucoma before vision is lost by examining the optic nerve through a dilated pupil and a visual field test. Vision loss resulting from damage to the optic nerve is irreversible but is preventable if detected early and treatment is started immediately.

If detected early, glaucoma is treatable with eye drops that lower the pressure in the eye. Treatment may include medication or surgery, both of which can have high success rates. If eye drops are not effective, medication can reduce the level of fluid in the eye, but it can produce side effects. Laser surgery is also used to regulate eye pressure.

Diabetic Retinopathy

Diabetic retinopathy is associated with diabetes, both type I (insulin dependent) and type II, frequently non-insulin-dependent. People with diabetes are at risk for losing vision from retinopathy, as well as from cataracts or glaucoma. About 40 percent of people with diabetes have at least mild retinopathy. Its incidence increases with the duration of the disease and when blood glucose levels cannot be controlled. Diabetic retinopathy results when small blood vessels stop feeding the retina properly. In the early stages, the blood vessels may leak fluid in the retina, which can affect the macula, the entire retina, or the vitreous, and can distort vision. In the later stages, new vessels may grow and send blood into the center of the eye, causing serious vision loss. Diabetic retinopathy results in poor vision for reading; print is distorted or blurred. Many people experience increased sensitivity to glare. Diabetes also increases the possibility of cataract.

Retinopathy associated with diabetes cannot be prevented although control of blood sugar levels and high blood pressure may often deter the progression of diabetic eye disease. If warning signs are present, visual problems associated with the condition can be prevented if eyes are examined at the earliest possible time. If the presence of blood in the vitreous does not resolve over time, a vitrectomy, or surgical removal of the vitreous, can be performed. Blood and scar tissue are removed from the eye, and the vitreous is replaced with a clear solution. In many cases, laser treatment can restore vision, stabilize it, or at least delay severe vision loss. A type of laser treatment called panretinal photocoagulation can seal off leaking vessels and destroy abnormal ones, when the leaking is caused by the growth of fragile new blood vessels.

If untreated, diabetic retinopathy can result in total blindness, so it is very important that older people with diabetes have an eye exam through dilated pupils every year. As mentioned earlier, individuals who are Hispanic, African-American, or Native American are at a greater risk of developing diabetes, so that individuals with these ethnic heritages should have routine annual medical and eye care.

Cataracts

Cataracts are cloudy areas in part or all of the lens of the eye. In a young person, the lens is crystal clear and allows light to pass through and focus on the retina. Cataracts prevent light from easily passing through the lens, and this causes loss of vision. Cataracts often form slowly and cause no pain, redness, or tearing in the eye. As the lens ages, the nucleus or center of the lens turns yellow and loses its ability to accommodate (focus for close work), although the lens usually remains clear. As the lens continues to age, the nucleus turns from yellow to amber and ultimately to brown. A cataract is not significant, however, until it interferes with vision. Although a cataract results in diminished acuity because of the opacification of the lens, it does not affect a particular portion of the field of vision but causes overall blurring. If a cataract becomes large or dense, it usually can be removed by surgery. Some cataracts stay small and do not change eyesight significantly.

Older people with cataracts experience decreased visual acuity, more difficulty seeing in poorly lit environments owing to a decrease in contrast sensitivity, increased sensitivity to light and glare. Print appears hazy and contrast is limited. Approximately 50 percent of Americans between ages 65 and 74, and 70 percent age 75 and over have cataracts (Faye, Rosenthal, & Sussman-Skalka, 1995).

Cataract surgery has a high success rate. Ninety-five percent of patients experience improved vision if no other eye conditions are present. During surgery, the doctor removes the clouded lens and, in most cases, inserts a clear intraocular lens of appropriate power. Cataract surgery is generally very safe. Complications do result from cataract surgery in approximately 5 percent of cases. It is one of the most common surgeries performed in the United States. Eyeglasses with thick lenses after surgery are no longer needed because of the implanted lens.

Vision Loss Resulting from Stroke

It is also important to mention that a cerebral stroke can cause vision loss. Just as a stroke may involve one side of the body, hemianopsia, a defect of the optic pathways in the brain, can result in vision loss in half of the visual field. Hemianopsia in either hemisphere can affect reading. The individual may have difficulty finding the beginning of lines of text if the vision loss is on the left; it may be difficult to see the ends of words if the vision loss is on the right. The individual may consistently bump into objects on the affected side and must learn to make good use of remaining vision associated with the unaffected hemisphere.

Low Vision

The specialization of low vision within optometry and ophthalmology has created greater awareness that although vision problems can hinder independent functioning, remaining vision can be utilized to continue productive activity. This is a critical message to convey. Many professionals, even in the ophthalmological community, need to be mindful of the critical role low vision rehabilitation can play in the lives of people with impaired vision. Being classified as having *low vision* is far less ominous than being told one is *blind* or *legally blind.* Older individuals and those with whom they come in contact are less frightened of the term low vision and are therefore more able to confront this level of vision loss. Societal fears and the myths about blindness have centered around total blindness. In large measure, age-related vision loss is not synonymous with total blindness but with low vision.

Many people with vision loss can enhance their visual functioning with the use of low vision devices. Low vision devices are optical devices that are stronger than regular eyeglasses and include microscopic and telescopic glasses, lenses that filter light, and magnifying glasses. There are also some useful electronic devices that can either be handheld or placed directly on the printed page. People with low vision often make good improvements in visual functioning through the use of low vision devices.

The Psychosocial Component of Age-Related Vision Loss

The impact of age-related vision loss can be enormous. (See Chapter 4 for additional discussion of these issues.) Many older people report that they had never really understood the impact just by hearing their contemporaries talk about vision problems—until it happened to them. In *Profiles in Aging and Vision* (Orr, 1998b) and in *The World Through Their Eyes* (Fangmeier, 1995) older people eloquently convey this message. A common emotion expressed by the older people in *Profiles* was "At first I was terrified. My children became even more terrified. Then I found out about services that are available to people like us . . . ." Nicolette Ringgold (1991), a university professor who becomes visually impaired as a result of macular degeneration, tells the story of how she identified services and creatively adapted to her own vision loss in *Out of the Corner of My Eye*.

A frequent reaction to deteriorating vision is the fear that the older person will not be able to continue to live alone, independently, within his or her own home and familiar community. The older person and family members alike think that a nursing home may be the only option. These beliefs occur primarily because older people and their family members are unaware that vision-related services exist and that these services can enable them to continue to function independently, with little or no assistance from others. Many fear that they will become completely dependent on others and that they will lose control over their lives, over their familiar environment.

One of the harshest realities is acknowledging that driving is no longer possible. For the older person, giving up driving usually represents a significant loss and signifies (or is synonymous with) giving up one's independence. When older people realize they cannot continue to perform a routine task confidently, they may discontinue that activity, no matter how valued or essential it is to their lives. These activities might include cooking, watching TV, or going to a religious service. When an older person realizes that additional assistance is needed, he or she wants the type of assistance to be something very "normal" and familiar, such as stronger lenses, not something different, such as a handheld magnifier.

Although many optical and nonoptical adaptive devices exist, some older people are resistant to using them (Orr, 1997). Using a different technique requires older people to accept that they are different from others and different from themselves at earlier stages of life. An internal struggle ensues. The older person may contemplate: Is it better to stay at home rather than walk around the neighborhood using a white cane? Is it better not to accept a dinner invitation or to read the restaurant menu with a lighted magnifier? In short, does using a device or adaptation represent the ability to continue to function independently, or does it feel like "giving in" to limitation and defeat? It could mean recognizing that one is aging at a time when there are solutions, scientific advances in medicine, ophthalmology, technology, and vision rehabilitation, and that taking advantage of what is available in spite of the fact that it is unfamiliar can make the difference between dependence and independence. The latter view requires a recognition that aging is another developmental stage of the life cycle, posing challenges and opportunities for further exploration and growth and, for many, doing old tasks in a new way. Without vision rehabilitation services, vision loss can be a socially and physically isolating situation.

Without question, vision loss is a family issue, and there is a growing need for vision rehabilitation to involve family members in the instruction and acquisition of adaptive skills and the use of adaptive equipment (see Chapter 7). Family members experience their own set of emotions and fears associated with an older person's vision loss. They struggle with whether or not to help, how to help, and when to help or not to help. A common reaction is to want to jump in and "do for" the older person whom they love, and the older person's safety is of paramount importance.

Family members, adult children in particular, looking for solutions frequently do not know where to start their search. Far too often, what family members think they should be looking for is "care" for the older person when they cannot be there—someone to be in the home, helping with tasks the older person can no longer do, making certain that their parent is safe and will not risk injury. Far less often do family members think about older people learning new ways to do things for themselves. Therefore, families may not think to seek vision rehabilitation services. Participation in a support group for the newly visually impaired person can play a critical role in helping older people adjust to the loss by meeting others experiencing similar reactions and day-to-day struggles. A support group is an invaluable source of information about the resources and services available. Support groups are also important for family members to help them understand how they can locate appropriate resources and facilitate the independent functioning of their loved ones.

Vision Rehabilitation Services

Rowe and Kahn (1997) propose the concept of *resilience,* the speed and completeness with which people recover from critical life events as an important determinant of successful aging. For older people experiencing age-related vision loss, access to vision rehabilitation services can make the difference between feeling dependent and feeling self-confident and self-reliant. The older person's sense of self-efficacy and self-worth are increased.

Vision rehabilitation services are provided by specially trained vision rehabilitation professionals. Rehabilitation teachers provide instruction in adaptive techniques for carrying out activities of daily living (ADLs, such as bathing, eating, dressing, and moving around the house) and instrumental activities of daily living (IADLs, such as preparing meals, shopping, and doing housework), teach indoor orientation to the environment, and make recommendations for modifications to the older person's physical environment to enhance independent functioning. Orientation and mobility (O&M) specialists teach outdoor orientation and instruction in the use of the long (white) cane. They can teach older people to negotiate their outdoor environment, to get to places of need and interest such as the grocery store or place of worship. They can also teach the older person to use public transit where it is available. Low vision therapists can teach older people how to successfully use optical devices such as magnification and telescopic devices prescribed by the low vision optometrist or ophthalmologist. Some professionals have training and expertise in all of these areas of vision rehabilitation and are called vision rehabilitation therapists.

The number of private and public agencies serving people with visual impairments, which respond to the needs of older people, has grown enormously over the last 20 years. In many cases, insufficient funding has been the major barrier for organizations serving this population. The vision rehabilitation service delivery system does not have the same level or degree of organizational structure as the aging network. The needs of older persons experiencing vision loss have not fit neatly into either the aging or the vision systems of services. As the population of people with vision problems shifted from the young to the 55 and older age groups, the largest portion of adults who were blind or visually impaired were not eligible for vocational rehabilitation services. But because an older person's life expectancy at 65 can be 20 or more years, productive activity, independent functioning, and ongoing contributions to family and community remain important goals. A brief history of the development of services for people who are blind or visually impaired sheds some light on why vision-related services for older people, although they do exist, are inadequate to meet the demands of this growing population.

The field of blindness and visual impairment has its roots in the education of blind children in the middle of the nineteenth century. Services for adults grew largely from the two World Wars when veterans who lost their vision in battle returned home. It was not until after World War II that vision rehabilitation services as we know them today became professionalized. Rehabilitation legislation has focused on vocational rehabilitation for the purpose of returning people to the world of work. The most significant legislation is the Rehabilitation Act of 1973 and its amendments to date. It is only as recently as 1986 that the first federal funding was allocated for independent living for older individuals who were blind or visually impaired under Title VII of the Rehabilitation Act.

Arduous legislative advocacy efforts have been the cornerstone of the development of vision rehabilitation services for older Americans. The first goal was to establish a separate portion of the Rehabilitation Act specifically for training in independent living skills for older blind and visually impaired persons; that became Title VII, Part C (now known as Title VII, Chapter 2) of the Act. The efforts to secure funding for independent living provided by Chapter 2 is truly the focus of the history of the development of vision rehabilitation services for older people. The second step was to operationalize Part C by appropriating funds for these independent living services (Rogers & Orr, 1999). The long-term goal has been to increase the funding level for Chapter 2, the only federal funding specifically targeted to serve this population, so that each state could have an equitable distribution of funds to match its population of older persons with impaired vision (Rogers & Orr, 1999).

During the last two reauthorizations of the Rehabilitation Act, advocates had to fight to preserve the integrity of the Chapter 2 program, against the trend toward provision of generic services by generalists not trained in the critical areas of rehabilitation teaching, O&M, and low vision instruction. Just as we have seen in education that even the most noble concept of mainstreaming children into the general classroom is not always the best educational environment and method for every child, generic services for adults cannot consistently include special instruction in braille, cane travel, and the use of adaptive equipment and other adaptive techniques of a highly specialized nature, particularly when the standard is a master's degree in rehabilitation teaching or O&M.

Each year, only a fraction of the newly visually impaired older population seeks and receives vision rehabilitation services. Five to seven years may pass from the onset of vision loss before older people seek services. In 1996, only 26,846 older individuals with visual impairments received vision rehabilitation services funded by Title VII, Chapter 2, of the Rehabilitation Act because of the program's limited funding level (Stephens, McBroom, & Lai, 1998). This represents only 1 percent of the older people eligible for services. In 1997, the American Foundation for the Blind's (AFB) National Aging and Vision

Network designed and implemented a National Advocacy Campaign to work toward the $13 million funding level that would trigger the transformation of Chapter 2 from a discretionary to a formula funding mechanism. The Fiscal Year (FY) 1999 Chapter 2 allocation was still only $11.1 million. As of the fall of 1999, $15 million was included in the budget for Title VII, Chapter 2 services for FY 2000. This action by Congress marks an important victory for advocates, but it does not diminish the need for continued efforts to promote the need for higher levels of funding.

CRITICAL ISSUES IN VISION REHABILITATION FOR OLDER AMERICANS

Essential to collaboration between professionals in the aging network and the vision rehabilitation field is an understanding of the critical issues facing vision rehabilitation today and in the near future. The following issues are important to both systems:

- ◆ The need for specialized services and specialized professionals
- ◆ The need to help older persons obtain productive activity
- ◆ The need for consumer empowerment and advocacy skills training
- ◆ The need to think of vision rehabilitation services as part of the continuum of home and community-based services
- ◆ Recognition and elimination of barriers that inhibit access to services

Specialized Services and Specialized Professionals

An understanding of the need for collaboration between the fields of vision and aging would not be complete without mention of the enormous advocacy efforts necessary to ensure the future of specialized services targeted to the needs of older individuals and delivered by professionals specifically trained to provide these services. For the most part, vision rehabilitation services have not traditionally been covered expenses through Medicare, Medicaid, or private insurance. The practice of vision-related rehabilitation grew out of an educational model, rather than a medical model, and the vision rehabilitation field has traditionally worked to remain outside the medical service delivery system, largely because it viewed its services as highly specialized but as not requiring the prescription of a physician. At present, however, there are neither sufficient funds nor personnel to meet the demand for services. (See Chapter 10 for a detailed discussion of this issue.)

Many complex issues relating to such areas as training, funding, and third-party reimbursement will need to be explored and resolved in the years ahead to ensure effective service delivery. For example, occupational therapists (OTs) are finding that large numbers of older persons being treated for a variety of physical rehabilitation needs are also visually impaired. Although the services provided by such practitioners are reimbursable through the health system, traditionally these professionals have not been trained in areas relating to low vision rehabilitation.

At the same time, professionals in vision rehabilitation are beginning to recognize that vision loss is a health care issue, along with the other physical and health conditions associated with aging, and many believe that it is both appropriate and necessary for vision-related services to be reimbursed through the health system. Reimbursement, however, often depends on certification and licensure requirements, and legislative and certification efforts are being undertaken.

Against the background of these fast-changing trends, the need for collaboration and appropriate service referral remains. For example, OTs, who see many older people in their routine OT practices, could become a referral source for these clients to vision rehabilitation services if they were fully aware of vision rehabilitation. An important goal for the vision field is to work collaboratively with OTs and other health professionals to mutually delineate the core curriculum needed by these practitioners to work in low vision rehabilitation and to decide where the role of one service provider ends and the vision rehabilitation professional (the RT or O&M specialist) begins.

Opportunities for Productive Activity

After three decades of struggle for federal funds to provide independent living services to older people who are blind or visually impaired, it is now time to focus attention on the issue of increased access to vocational rehabilitation services for older people that would enable older employees to remain in the workforce and older retirees to reenter the workforce if they desire. This is probably one of the hardest issues that the vision rehabilitation field has ever tackled. Although more attention is being given to the value of the older worker than ever before, media coverage makes it clear that seasoned workers in their 50s continue to be downsized, while younger, more technically savvy and less expensive employees are hired.

This situation makes it a considerable challenge to educate employers that mature workers, individuals in their 50s and early 60s who begin to have vision problems, can remain effective employees through vocational rehabilitation services. It is especially important that young older people do not unnecessarily select early retirement. Reentering the workforce is a challenge for everyone, perhaps especially for the older person who is visually impaired.

To create opportunities for remunerative employment for middle-aged and older workers, the vision rehabilitation field also must look within itself. Vocational rehabilitation counselors and other professionals who assess the older consumer's rehabilitation goals need to seriously consider the individual's employment potential. They must include vocational rehabilitation as one of the older person's possible rehabilitation goals. For too long, rehabilitation professionals have struggled over this issue, recognizing all the barriers to achieving success for the older consumer in the area of vocational rehabilitation and employment. No matter how difficult, these professionals must challenge themselves first before they can be convincing to employers (Miller, 1991).

Productive activity is an extremely important issue in gerontology and must not be overlooked in relation to older people who are visually impaired. The term encompasses a broad range of activities in addition to paid employment, including volunteerism, caring for and maintaining a household, family caregiving, and caring for neighbors or peers. Most older people are in fact productive; they make contributions mostly in the form of informal supports to others and volunteer work. Informal help to friends and relatives is common between the ages of 55 and 64 and remains significant to age 75 and even beyond. Older visually impaired persons can be included in this description. Visual impairment need not be an impediment to productive activity and the older person's self-perception as a contributing member of the family or community. Professionals can be creative in developing volunteer opportunities as well as opportunities for the older individual who is visually impaired to assume mentoring and leadership roles.

Consumer Empowerment and Advocacy Skills Training

Choice is contingent on having and understanding options. Information is empowerment. Many older people with visual impairments and their family members still do not have the information they need to make informed decisions about steps to address deteriorating vision. Even when connected to the vision rehabilitation system, many do not find out about all the services available to them. Thus, an important, yet underaddressed, independent living skill is the need to teach advocacy strategies to older people as part of rehabilitation services so that consumers become informed and empowered to assume control over decisions affecting their lives.

Older people also can serve as tremendous resources to agencies serving people who are blind or visually impaired by serving on advisory committees and task forces and participating in program planning. Older people with visual impairments participating in consumer focus groups around the country found that effective service delivery depends on the following critical elements, including consumer involvement (Crews, 1996):

◆ Consumer involvement in all phases of planning and delivering of services
◆ An understanding that older people with impaired vision are clients of both the aging and vision service delivery systems
◆ Collaboration among service providers to ensure comprehensive and holistic rehabilitation and supportive services and to maximize scarce resources on behalf of consumers.

Vision Rehabilitation Services as Part of Home- and Community-Based Services

It is important for professionals in the vision field and the aging network to conceptualize vision rehabilitation services as part of home- and community-based long-term services—programs that provide the range of services that enable older people to continue to remain in their own homes and function as independently as possible. Both communities are similar in philosophy and in their operations, and both have the goals of promoting independence and quality of life. Both home- and community-based services and vision rehabilitation services focus on functional assessment and the services required to improve functioning.

Because two-thirds of older persons who are severely visually impaired also have at least one other serious chronic disability or illness, many of these individuals qualify for home- and community-based services on the basis of their impairment in performing ADLs. For them, the concern is whether program outreach, communication, needs assessment, care management, and other services are carried out in ways that accommodate their vision loss. Thus, inclusion of vision-related rehabilitation services in a home- and community-based long-term services package would not only increase the independence of older people who are visually imparied but also reduce their need for ongoing supportive services.

Barriers to Services

We need to acknowledge that serious barriers to vision-related rehabilitation services still exist. Barriers include attitudinal as well as economic, geographic, language, and cultural obstacles. Societal values determine the priority of resource allocation. The Americans with Disabilities Act has helped; universal design needs to increasingly consider the needs of people who are blind or visually impaired.

Myths and stereotypic perceptions about blindness and people who are blind have endured throughout the twentieth century, including unrealistic ideas of blind people as either all-knowing seers to be revered or as beggars to be pitied. Even now, some people still describe an individual who is blind and able to do routine activities as "amazing" and "phenomenal." Until the general public understands that someone who is blind or visually impaired is capable of doing the same activities as people in the mainstream and knows something about how this is possible, societal perceptions and attitudes will remain inaccurate.

Societal values and attitudes about older Americans in general reveal great bias. Ageism remains a powerful force in America and can often be seen in the legislative and political arena. Activity and productivity levels are directly related to whether we perceive an older person as "old" (Kahn, 1986). These negative attitudes about the abilities of both aging and visually impaired individuals, as well as lack of specific information about vision rehabilitation services, may prevent visually impaired older people themselves, family and friends, and even the professionals who assist them from knowing about or attempting to obtain the services that can maximize their independent living. The greater the level of activity, the younger an elder appears. Thus, the responsibility rests within the vision field and aging network to educate both professionals and the general public about the capabilities of people who are both visually impaired and older. And, because many of the barriers to obtaining vision rehabilitation services are attitudinal in nature, education and outreach services are crucial, both to the general public and particularly to older people in high-risk groups and in areas with limited access to services.

INTO THE NEW MILLENNIUM

At least since the time when Robert Butler (1975) coined the term *ageism*, American society has been aware of the negative images of aging—the post-retirement years characterized by symptoms of deteriorating health, increasing limitations in physical and cognitive functioning, and lack of productive activity. In a recent significant contribution to the gerontological literature, Rowe & Kahn (1998) include engagement in life as one of the three components of successful aging along with avoiding disease and maintaining high cognitive and physical function. Gerontology continues to broaden its perspective of aging from its earlier concern with disease and disability to a more active and energized view of aging that includes the concept of successful aging, transforming our thinking about the quality of life that is possible to achieve and sustain as Americans age. Older people who are blind or visually impaired must be included in that conceptualization.

The fight for additional funding for Chapter 2 has been ongoing since it was legislated through the 1978 amendments to the Rehabilitation Act, leading to its first funding in 1986 and the campaign continues for the year 2000 budget.

A National Agenda on Vision and Aging

American society is faced with the task of planning for the new millennium and the next cohorts of older people experiencing age-related vision loss. The United States has been experiencing the economic, social, and health care consequences of a burgeoning aging population. Congress continually debates whether this country can afford today's and tomorrow's elderly. Some of the largest challenges that affect all Americans include Social Security and Medicare reform, long-term care, and tax credits for family caregivers.

A National Agenda on Vision and Aging is needed to guide us through the 21st century. The National Aging and Vision Network, a network of more than 300 organizations, vision professionals, and older visually impaired consumers, organized and convened by the American Foundation for the Blind, has developed such an agenda.

The purpose of the National Agenda on Vision and Aging is to shape public policies and public attitudes that enable individuals age 55 and older who are blind or visually impaired to participate fully in all aspects of society. The following goals are a focal point for mobilizing collective action in the years ahead:

1. Develop self-advocacy awareness and skills of older persons who are blind or visually impaired and their family members.
2. Increase public awareness and promote positive attitudes about the needs and capabilities of older individuals who are blind or visually impaired.
3. Increase the availability of and access to vision rehabilitation services through adequate public funding.
4. Increase the supply of qualified personnel to meet the needs of older persons who are blind or visually impaired.
5. Expand access to information and community resources such as transportation and employment.
6. Promote the coordination of data collection and outcome measurement efforts that support the targeted goals of increased consumer self-advocacy, greater public awareness of vision rehabilitation services, sufficient funding for services, an increased supply of qualified personnel, and expanded access to information and community resources.
7. Position the vision rehabilitation field for health system reimbursement.

Role of the Aging Network

Professionals in the aging network can play a vital role in ensuring that their older consumers who are blind or visually impaired have access to the services they need. For example, the aging network can join in the advocacy efforts to expand funding for Title VII, Chapter 2. In 1999, one State Unit on Aging added Chapter 2 to its legislative advocacy agenda, recognizing that not only Older Americans Act funds, Social Security, and Medicare were necessary, but also the vision rehabilitation funds were needed through the Rehabilitation Act for their consumers. We hope the action of this one state unit will set a trend for others across the country. Professionals in the aging network also can support the National Agenda on Vision and Aging by working hand-in-hand with their colleagues in the vision field to achieve the Agenda's goals.

Professionals in the aging network also can include questions about vision loss and visual functioning in their consumer needs assessment instruments and can include partnership with the vision rehabilitation field at the state and local levels in the annual state plans. Because older individuals with impaired vision need services from more than solely the vision rehabilitation field, it is essential that professionals across many disciplines work collaboratively to ensure that they receive comprehensive and holistic services. Much of the attention in the aging field is on the care of the enormous number of older people with functional impairments in ADLs and IADLs. As noted by Clark (1997), collaboration among different professionals will take on greater importance as geriatric care moves "increasingly into the realm of quality of life and not simply life extension." Collaboration needs to be developed among professionals within a field, among professionals across many disciplines, and among organizations and service delivery systems.

The vision rehabilitation field alone cannot champion the needs of older people who are visually impaired. The aging network and allied health professionals also need to join the cause, because these older people represent our mutual concern and our society's future.

REFERENCES

Administration on Aging (1998). *Profile of older Americans, 1998.* Washington, DC: U.S. Department of Health and Human Services.

Butler, R. (1975). *Why survive: Being old in America.* New York: Harper and Row.

Clark, P. G. (1997). Values in health care professional socialization: Implications for geriatric education in interdisciplinary teamwork. *The Gerontologist, 37* (4), 441–451.

Crews, J. E. (1996). *Critical concerns and effective practices: Final focus group report*. New York: The Lighthouse Inc.

Duffy, M. A., & Beliveau-Toby, M. (1991). *New independence for older persons with vision loss in long-term care facilities*. Mohegan Lake, NY: AWARE.

Fangmeier, R. (1995). *The world through their eyes (videotape)*. New York: The Lighthouse Inc.

Faye, E., Rosenthal, B., & Sussman-Skalka, C. (1995). *Cataract and the aging eye*. New York: The Lighthouse National Center for Vision and Aging.

Griffin-Shirley, N., & Orr, A. L. (1993). *Aging and vision loss: Guidelines for an innovative personnel preparation curriculum in gerontology*. New York: AFB Press.

Kahn, R. L. (1986). Productive activities and well being. Paper presented at the annual meeting of The Gerontological Society of America, Chicago, IL.

Miller, G. (1991). Don't burn my boats without my permission. In N. Weber (Ed.), *Vision and aging: Issues in social work practice*. New York: Haworth Press, pp. 57–68.

National Advisory Eye Council (1993). *Vision research: A national plan, 1994–1998*. Bethesda, MD: National Eye Institute, National Institutes of Health.

Orr, A. L. (1992a). The psychosocial aspects of aging and vision. In N. Weber (Ed.)., *Vision and aging issues in social work practice*. New York: Haworth Press, pp. 1–14.

Orr, A. L. (1992b). *Vision and aging: Crossroads to service delivery*. New York: AFB Press.

Orr, A. L. (1997). Assistive technologies for older persons who are visually impaired. In R. Lubinski, & D. J. Higginbotham (Eds.), *Communication technologies for the elderly: Vision, hearing and speech*. San Diego: Singular, pp. 71–102.

Orr, A. L. (1998a). *Issues in aging and vision: A curriculum for university programs and in-service training*. New York: AFB Press.

Orr, A. L. (1998b). *Profiles in aging and vision* (videotape). New York: AFB Press.

Ringgold, N. P. (1991). *Out of the corner of my eye: Living with vision loss in later life*. New York: American Foundation for the Blind.

Rogers, P., & Orr, A. L. (1999). *History of efforts to establish a national service delivery program for older people who are blind or visually impaired*. Review, 31(3), 103–112.

Rogers, P., & Orr, A. L. (2000). Current issues and future directions in the field of aging and vision. In B. Silverstone, M. Lang, B. Rosenthal & E. Faye (Eds.), *The Lighthouse handbook on vision impairment and vision rehabilitation*. New York: Oxford University Press.

Rowe, J. W., & Kahn, R. L. (1997). Successful aging. *The Gerontologist, 37* (4), 433–440.

Rowe, J. W., & Kahn, R. L. (1998). *Successful aging.* New York: Random House.

Schmeidler E., & Halfmann, D. (1997). Estimated rates of visual impairment among older Americans by State, 1995. Unpublished data. American Foundation for the Blind.

Schmeidler, E., & Halfmann, D. (1998). Vision of nursing home residents; expected years of healthy life; and risk factors for adolescents. Demographic update. *Journal of Visual Impairment and Blindness, 92* (3), 221–224.

Spector, W. D., & Fleishman, J. A. (1998). Combining activities of daily living with instrumental activities of daily living to measure functional disability. *Journal of Gerontology, 53b* (1), 546–557.

Stephens, B., McBroom, L. W., & Lai, S. (1998). *Independent living services for older individuals who are blind, Title VII-Chapter 2 Annual Report for FY 1996.* Mississippi State, MS: MSU Rehabilitation Research and Training Center on Blindness and Low Vision.

PART TWO

Multidisciplinary Perspectives on Aging and Vision Loss

CHAPTER 4

Vision Care for Elderly Individuals: Innovation and Advancement in Low Vision Services

Alfred A. Rosenbloom, Jr.

Even though today's greater life expectancy is often accompanied by a higher incidence of ocular and degenerative disorders, there has also been an increase in literacy among aging persons. A greater number of these individuals are unwilling to accept poor vision as a natural consequence of advancing age and are demanding that more attention be given to comprehensive health care. For optometry, providing adequate vision care for aging patients with low vision is a continuing challenge to professional skills and knowledge. Low vision is broadly defined as a visual impairment not correctable by standard eyeglasses, contact lenses, medicine, or surgery that interferes with the ability of the individual to perform everyday activities. This challenge gives rise to four important questions:

1. What are contemporary concepts of low vision and aging that may serve as a frame of reference for understanding the provision of low vision care for elderly individuals?
2. What are the most common eye diseases associated with visual impairment of the aging?

3. What are the essential understandings about the nature of an aging person's visual impairment as it relates to the total process of rehabilitation?
4. What new directions in research and development are needed to maximize low vision patient care?

CONTEMPORARY CONCEPTS OF AGING AND LOW VISION

Developing an understanding of certain basic contemporary concepts relating to aging, low vision, and low vision rehabilitation will help to establish a frame of reference for examining the provision of low vision services to the elderly segment of the population.

Aging

The burgeoning of the elderly population has been extensively described. In the year 2000, 35 million people will be 65 or older, and by 2030, one in five persons will be over the age of 65 (AARP, 1991). By definition, aging describes the physiological changes in a person's life from one point in time to another, the adjustment of human beings to their environment between maturity and death. Aging is a continuous process and, although developmental in nature, it is highly individualized, especially in the area of health problems. Old age can mean different things to different people.

The demographic revolution is illustrated in everyday clinical practice, where there are increasing numbers of the young-old (65–75) and old-old (75–85), and more and more in that rapidly growing sector, the oldest-old (over 85).

Older persons constitute the most vulnerable group for such age-related eye disorders as cataracts, macular degeneration, glaucoma, and diabetic retinopathy. And, as increasing numbers of individuals live well into their 80s and 90s, both the numbers and percentage of older persons with vision impairments will increase. The National Center for Health Statistics (Nelson, 1987) reports that most people experiencing visual impairment are age 65 and over; some 3.3 million people have some difficulty seeing or are legally blind in one or both eyes. This composite number includes 9.5 percent of the population between the ages of 65 and 74, 16 percent between the ages of 75 and 84, and 26 percent of age 85 and older. Many of these individuals are living with families, foster families, and friends. In fact, there are five elderly widows for every elderly widower. One-half of all women over 75 live alone.

Documenting the presence of multiple impairments among elderly persons, researchers report increases with age in chronic health conditions such as hearing loss, arthritis, high blood pressure, heart conditions, and orthopedic impairments. See Chapters 2 and 5. These impairments are only part of the difficulties visually impaired elderly people cope with; there are also psychological and social issues. Problems commonly associated with the aging process may include separation from family members, the loss of a spouse, withdrawal from earlier life roles, retirement, a decrease in overall income, and the loss of family and friends. The onset of vision loss exacerbates the other problems that are associated with attempts to maintain an independent lifestyle.

It is important to remember that there are normal aging changes taking place in visual function for the person over age 60. Such normal phenomena as reduced visual activity, refractive state changes involving increased hyperopia (farsightedness) or myopia (nearsightedness) and astigmatic shifts, steadily decreasing powers of accommodation to differing viewing distances, decreased rate of dark adaptation and decreased resistance to glare lead to increased difficulty for elderly persons in coping adequately with their visual environment. For the eye to see an image or object, light must pass through the cornea and lens and be focused on the retina. Related physiological changes involve thickening of the lens, increased entoptic light scatter, resulting from diffuse transmission of light through the sclera and iris; flares produced at various refractive (light-bending) surfaces; specular reflections; and scatter within the ocular media due to a loss of homogeneity in the structure of the lens and vitreous. (See Figure 1 for a diagram of the eye and a description of its major structures.) There is also a general reduction in pupillary diameter in both the dark- and light-adapted eye as a function of age.

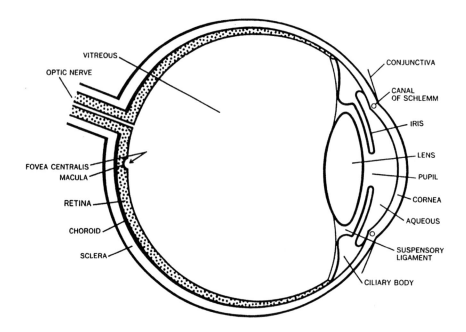

Cornea: The transparent part of the outer layer situated in front of the eyeball, responsible for helping to focus light

Sclera: The tough, white, outermost layer that protects the eye

Choroid: The middle layer of the eye that contains the network of blood vessels that nourish the eye

Iris: The round, colored part of the eye opens and closes to regulate the amount of light that enters the eye

Pupil: The round opening in the center of the iris that constricts and enlarges in response to light and helps focus light on the retina

Lens: The transparent structure behind the iris that changes its shape to bring rays of light to focus on the retina

Aqueous: A water fluid that fills the portion of the eye in front of the lens

Vitreous: The clear gel that fills and supports the eyeball

Retina: The innermost layer of the eye where light comes into focus and containing nerve cells and fibers that extend from the eye to the visual cortex of the brain

Macula: The central area of the retina that is responsible for fine visual tasks

Fovea centralis: The central point on the retina where light rays come together and visual acuity is greatest

Figure 1
Cross section of the eye

Source: Prevent Blindness America.

Low Vision

Low vision may be considered as the middle range of a continuum of impairment of visual function, from normal vision to total blindness. In low vision there is a reduction in visual activity or visual field, or both, in which vision cannot be significantly improved by conventional eyeglasses, and the loss of vision substantially interferes with learning processes, vocational or avocational pursuits, social interactions, or the activities of daily living. This functional, multidisciplinary conception of visual ability is in marked contrast to the still prevailing use in various quarters of the definition of legal blindness, which is categorized as 20/200 or worse visual acuity in the better seeing eye or a visual field that, in its widest diameter, does not exceed 20 degrees. Even individuals with the same clinical vision may have different visual capabilities and see very differently. Such a definition tells nothing about a person's ability to see or to function visually, since it conveys no information about visual efficiency, near or reading vision, nature and extent of the visual field, motility skills, binocular function, general intelligence, overall maturity, or personal motivation. A functional emphasis concerned with the individual and his or her ability to perform essential or desirable tasks dictates a holistic, multidisciplinary approach to vision care.

The ninth revision of the *International Classification of Diseases* of the World Health Organization (1978) includes codes for both blindness and low vision. This classification broadly defines blindness as having no vision or no significant usable vision. Low vision is also defined as having a significant visual impairment, but also having significant usable residual vision. These new definitions recognize the debilitating effects of a loss in contrast sensitivity, increased light scatter from a turbid ocular media, changes in dark adaptation, spectral sensitivity, and perceptual complications from the use of high magnification. In addition, these definitions are superior to the traditional criteria, which use only visual acuity or visual field restrictions as a quantitative determination. They are, of necessity, broad and nonspecific about visual acuity levels or other visual functions, because of the determination of what is significant, usable vision depends not only on clinical data, but also, in a large measure, on the circumstances of an individual's life. Individual adaptations to changes in visual functioning are affected by the nature and extent of the vision loss, whether it is stable or progressive, and the presence of other problems influencing the person's ability to cope with the demands of daily living.

For the low vision patient, many of the "normal" aging changes are exacerbated, depending on the nature and effect of the ocular and, not infrequently, the systemic disease processes. It is important to know not only the degree of visual impairment with age, but also the effect of these visual decrements on the adaptive behavior of the individual. From a behavioral standpoint, some reductions in visual acuity, color vision, and depth perception might not result in significant personal handicaps that have important social consequences. It is particularly true in situations in which the onset of the visual impairment is gradual and some compensation is made by using low vision devices, by developing other skills, and by making changes in the environment.

Low Vision Rehabilitation

Low vision rehabilitation is a process comprising a range of services directed in a coordinated manner toward helping the person with low vision achieve fulfilling and realizable goals in those activities affected by the visual loss. These services may include, but are not limited to, medical, optometric, social, vocational, rehabilitative, and psychological services. Our concern is to care for the geriatric patient with impaired vision so that he or she may attain valued activities, a degree of self-sufficiency, emotional independence, and satisfaction in social interactions with others. Too often our goals are physical in nature and overlook these emotional, intellectual, and social aspects of living.

COMMON EYE DISEASES ASSOCIATED WITH AGING AND VISUAL IMPAIRMENT

Even when people are healthy and seek and receive regular appropriate eye care, they are likely to experience the effects of some normal changes in their eyes and vision as they grow older. These normal or expected changes have a subtle effect on how well an older person sees. (Readers can refer to Figure 1 for specific structures of the eye referred to in the discussions of common eye diseases.) The optic nerve carries the message to the brain for interpretation. Normal changes that occur during aging reduce the amount or quality of light that passes through the eye. In understanding the four major diseases associated with aging and visual impairment, it is helpful to examine several diagrams of the eye, with particular attention to a cross-sectional view. It is also important to define the major components of the eye (see Figure 1).

The four eye diseases that are the primary causes of visual impairment in elderly people are cataracts, diabetic retinopathy, glaucoma, and age-related macular degeneration. It is not uncommon for older people to experience more than one of these conditions, either consecutively or simultaneously.

Cataracts

Cataract is defined as a painless, progressive clouding of the lens of the eye. The condition usually develops in only one eye at a time, and the degree of impairment can vary greatly among individuals. Fortunately, most people are not affected to the point of significant visual disability. For many, vision may be significantly enhanced.

It is not known how cataracts form. Basically, the opacity is caused by some change in the internal structure of the lens in which lens fibers coagulate and lens protein becomes insoluble and opaque. A further change in lens transparency may occur when water accumulates. Also, water may accumulate between the lens fibers. If the opacity progresses and the lens becomes opaque, the condition is referred to as a "mature" cataract. At that point, vision is markedly decreased.

The treatment for cataracts is removal of the lens. This is a safe surgical procedure that is usually performed under local anesthesia. The ophthalmologist removes the clouded lens and, in most cases, replaces it with an intraocular implant or artificial lens. The complication rate is low, and the majority of patients report improved vision.

Diabetic Retinopathy

Diabetic retinopathy is a condition that appears to some degree in most people who have had diabetes mellitus for at least 15 years. It almost always affects both eyes. Diabetes is better controlled today and patients live longer. Notwithstanding more effective control of blood sugar levels, there is increased frequency of diabetic retinopathy among older persons with long-established diabetes. Individuals may lessen the severity of retinal damage by following prescribed regimens carefully, particularly in regard to diet and exercise. The actual pathology of retinopathy is seen as microaneurysms, or small hemorrhages, and yellow-white exudates. As abnormal new blood vessels are formed, they may leak fluid, and consequently distort vision. Although there is no cure for diabetic retinopathy, the use of drugs may remove exudates, and photocoagulation by laser surgery helps to close new and leaky blood vessels.

Glaucoma

Glaucoma is a condition in which elevated intraocular pressure results in loss of the visual field and damage to the optic nerve. The formation of intraocular pressure is a complex process. The aqueous humor, the watery fluid between the cornea and the lens of the eye, is formed in the posterior chamber behind the iris and then circulates through the pupil into the anterior chamber. Here it is drained through the canal of Schlemm at the angle between the rim of the iris and the back of the cornea. The balance between the secretion and the outflow of this fluid, which nourishes the cornea and the lens, determines intraocular pressure. An increase in the pressure can result in compressed blood vessels within the eyeball, thereby depriving the retina of an adequate blood supply, resulting in impaired vision and even blindness.

The most common form of primary glaucoma affecting about 1 percent of people over age 40 is referred to as *chronic simple (open-angle) glaucoma*. The condition is generally without symptoms until late in its course; infrequently, however, blurred vision, not correctable with lenses, or complaints of a halo effect around lights may be the first signs of a problem. Therefore, the routine measurement of intraocular pressure every 1 or 2 years after age 35 is recommended for everyone, but especially for people with a family history of glaucoma and for persons of African-American ancestry.

Treatment for open-angle glaucoma usually involves medication to lower intraocular pressure. Pressure can be reduced by increasing aqueous outflow with miotics, drugs that cause the pupil of the eye to contract, or by decreasing aqueous formation with carbonic anhydrase inhibitors or beta-blocking agents. If this treatment fails, a drainage pathway through the trabecular meshwork can be created with laser surgery or by conventional glaucoma surgical techniques.

The less common form of primary glaucoma is *closed-angle glaucoma*. The condition results from intermittent contact of the iris and the inner surface of the trabecular meshwork with a consequent obstruction of the outflow of aqueous fluid. The result is an acute crisis in which the pressure within the eyeball rises suddenly. The attack is often accompanied by pain around the eye, headache, nausea, and vomiting. Immediate treatment with appropriate medication given within hours is necessary to relieve the pressure. Once the eye is stabilized, surgery is often performed to correct the reduced angle and to restore the free flow of aqueous fluid within the eye chamber.

Macular Degeneration

Age-related macular degeneration can actually occur at any age but is most common in elderly people. This condition is the most common cause of visual impairment among elderly persons.

There are two basic types of age-related maculopathy—dry and wet. In the dry type of the disease, aging yellow spots, called Drusen, are present with or without atrophy of the nerve fibers of the macular region. In this dry form, the visual acuity is usually not drastically affected. In the wet form, abnormal blood vessels "leak," hence the term wet. These vessels grow behind the retina in the subretinal space, and leak blood and fluid. With time, these blood vessels proliferate and grow into a scar. Once the scar has formed, there is no treatment, except for low vision rehabilitation, as the scar is the end result of this process.

Although the dry form of the disease is the most common, most irreversible vision loss is due to the wet form. It has been stated that approximately 10 to 15 percent of patients have the wet form, which is responsible for approximately ninety percent of severe vision loss from age-related maculopathy (Kanski, 1999).

The macula is at the center of the fovea centralis, the most sensitive spot for visual acuity within the retina. Thus, the most common symptoms of macular degeneration are a progressive loss of reading vision and of sharp distance vision, usually in both eyes. Distortion of details in the environment, waviness, or a smudge-like area in the central vision are common complaints.

Because the macular area degenerates in this disease, central vision is eventually lost, even though peripheral, or side, vision is maintained. Although the cause of this degeneration is unknown, the process is believed to be associated with a sclerosis of the choroidal blood vessels that supply nutrients to the macula area. Treatment for the condition has not been remarkably successful, although laser coagulation treatment in selected cases (approximately 13 percent of the cases) may slow or stabilize the progress of the disease if it is started soon enough. Low vision devices are especially successful in restoring, in most cases, some degree of improved residual vision especially at the reading distance.

VISUAL IMPAIRMENT IN ELDERLY PERSONS AND THE REHABILITATION PROCESS

A basic understanding of the nature of visual impairment in elderly persons will aid the practitioner in determining the type of low vision testing and the kinds of low vision devices to consider. Lubinas (1980) and others have noted that to develop a broad understanding of the visual performance characteristics of low vision patients, a differentiation must be made between two broad categories—optical effects and neural effects.

Optical Effects

Optical effects relate primarily to the physical structure of the eye. For example, a patient with an optically reduced visual loss resulting from irregularities in the refractive surfaces, such as the cornea or the lens, will usually suffer from a degradation of the visual image. This effect is characterized by lower visual acuity and reduced contrast sensitivity. Cunningham and Johnston's (1980) preliminary research results suggest that detection of low-contrast objects (such as steps, pavements, and different textures) is the critical visual task for safe pedestrian mobility.

With increased intraocular scatter and absorption of light by the media, higher than normal luminance levels are necessary. Consequently, such factors as low light levels in an individual's environment, poorly designed light fixtures, dimly lit passageways, and shadows surrounding objects result in reduced visual performance.

Neural Effects

Neural losses, regardless of origin, affect structures within the neural pathway and are most commonly expressed as a visual field defect, or loss of vision in some part of the individual's field of vision. A large percentage of the low vision patient population typically exhibits a reduction in visual acuity, or sharpness of vision. Reduced vision may result from a loss of vision in the center of the visual field. Reduced vision may also be complicated by metamorphopsia (a distorted perceptual image), a lowered contrast sensitivity, a poor tolerance to variations in luminance, and a dependence on high luminance levels. All these factors contribute to poor mobility, even if the peripheral visual field is intact.

Another neural effect relates to the size and extent of scotomas, or blind spots. This results in a loss of retinal sensitivity as only objects of sufficient size, illuminance, or contrast will be recognized. If these scotomas are numerous, the person may have increasing difficulty in interpreting visual information, to the point that some persons, despite relatively good visual acuity, are unable to read, even with magnification assistance. This effect may be likened to the crowding phenomenon reported by some people with amblyopia, in which letters are seen, but cannot be interpreted.

Although not as common as central visual field loss, people with vision loss in the peripheral visual field represent a significant group within the low vision population. People with peripheral visual field losses, along with poor dark adaptation, require high levels of light for travel mobility and detection of potential environmental hazards.

Vision changes also reduce an elderly person's ability to adapt appropriately when going from bright to dark surroundings. Poor adaptation to the dark leads to problems in walking or driving at night. This problem is often compounded by a reduced sense of balance, falling, and fear of falling. The importance of recognizing potential hazards in the person's domestic environment cannot be overemphasized. Difficulties in adapting to vision loss can be minimized by ensuring that there is adequate artificial and natural lighting and that such hazards as loose banisters, worn steps, torn linoleum, loose rugs, and highly polished floors are avoided or eliminated.

Psychological State

In addition to optical effects and neural effects, other factors influence a patient's performance during a vision examination. One of these factors is the psychological state of both patient and practitioner.

The patient may arrive for the examination in a state of high excitement, with unachievable expectations and unbridled hope, creating a heightened desire to be super helpful and to make the right decision. As a consequence, the patient is sometimes unreliable. In contrast, since for many older people vision loss has an adventitious onset, the aging person may still be in the throes of a kind of grief reaction to the loss. Such a reaction is usually characterized by confusion, self-pity, doubt, and reduced self-confidence, which may lead the patient to respond in an examination with slower, often inexact answers, apparent disinterest, and even submissiveness. The most helpful mindset is for the patient to be ready and eager to help, but with the understanding that seeking restoration of his or her former vision without limitations is not the goal.

Conversely, the practitioner must also be aware of his or her own reactions. It is extremely important that the identification of the patient's expressed and perceived needs, the collection of clinical data, and the development of the agreed-on plan of action must be paced to the skill, understanding, and psychological state of the patient at that particular time. Mehr and Fried (1975) note that sometimes "a program of masterful inactivity is preferable to an expensive aid."

Elderly patients seem to be relatively neglected in the provision of low vision services. There are a number of possible explanations for this observation related to the psychological set of both patient and practitioner:

1. Many of the elderly tend to accept gradual loss of vision as one of the inevitable consequences of growing older. As a result, they fail to seek appropriate help for their increasing visual disability.
2. Motivation is often lacking because the person does not understand that low vision devices can only facilitate the use of residual vision by improving blurred or distorted visual images; they cannot provide or restore vision.
3. Elderly patients with seriously impaired vision often do not communicate effectively with practitioners about their needs.
4. Practitioners frequently assume that elderly patients are not as capable of rehabilitation as more youthful persons. Consequently, elderly patients are not offered the full variety and range of services that are available.
5. Practitioners may feel they are examining patients too late in the process of a disease to permit optimal treatment and prevention of disability.

Vision Examination and Prescribing

Another basic factor in understanding visual impairment in older people is the importance of the quality and scope of the case history as recorded by the practitioner. Indeed, the outcome of the rehabilitation service is often dependent on this evaluative component. The most important factors for the practitioner to establish from the evaluative case history are the elderly patients' special needs or desires, their ability to adapt to new situations, their motivation to learn new visual habits, and their understanding of the uses and limitations of the low vision devices they will be using.

If an elderly patient has lived with his or her family and has sighted persons around him or her, efforts may be directed to finding devices that will allow him or her to participate in normal family activities, such as watching television, playing cards, sewing, and playing games. If the individual lives alone, however, more attention may be focused on specific and necessary tasks such as reading mail, identifying labels on medicine bottles or canned goods, and the activities that every person can enjoy.

Following a thorough case history and comprehensive low vision examination, the low vision specialist prescribes appropriate refractive and magnification systems. There are a variety of low vision devices, which may be hand-held, or stand magnifiers, or spectacle-mounted systems worn by the user. Corrections of greatest value to elderly patients include the use of hand-held and stand magnifiers that can be used at varying distances to increase the size of the image; the occasional use of spectacle-mounted or hand-held compact telescopic systems for viewing objects at a distance; high power reading additions; and microscopic-type reading lenses that are used close to the eye for near activities. In addition, closed circuit television systems (CCTVs) use a video camera to display an enlarged image of the material to be viewed on a television screen.

It is also important for the low vision practitioner to prescribe appropriate nonoptical aids such as large-print books, synthesized speech aids (such as talking clocks and calculators), illumination aids, talking books (recorded materials), cassette recorders, digital watches, reading stands, the use of blank cards or typoscopes made of black cardboard with a small window for viewing words to enhance print contrasts, heavily lined writing paper, and a myriad of other devices that can be used in the home and on the job.

Learning to Use the Appropriate Low Vision Devices

Use of low vision devices requires considerable adjustment and adaptive training. With increasing levels of magnification, there may be an associated decrease in the field of view, the working distance, or in both factors. Increasing levels of magnification may also result in smaller depth of focus, increased peripheral distortions, and aberrations. A notable exception is the CCTV, which can provide a high level of magnification at remote viewing distances with an adequate field of view.

The low vision patient will require supervised adaptive training in order to build and sustain motivation on visual tasks involving material and activities of interest to the patient. If rehabilitation is to be a success, extensive instruction in the use of low vision devices also requires retraining of old skills and teaching of new ones. There are various types of adaptive training, but the most frequent relate to reading, including discrimination of parts of or single words, recognition of these word elements, and integration to give meaning to these symbols.

In learning to use a low vision device whether spectacle, hand-held or stand magnifier, telemicroscope, or CCTV, there also are differences in establishing the correct working or focal distance for the lens. With increasing levels of magnification, the ability to move from word to word on one line and to find the next line without peripheral cues or scanning becomes increasingly difficult. Adapting to these differences may require starting with a weaker lens and using larger print in order to make the patient feel more secure and then easing gradually into using the maximum power.

To facilitate this adaptive process, it may be appropriate to utilize the loan system of devices, which allow a patient to become gradually used to the effects of greater magnification. This process emphasizes the need for continuing reassessment, supervision, and counseling as the patient exhibits frustration and develops new needs. This type of adaptive training, is, at times, more important than the provision of the low vision device itself.

Adaptive training for a person with low vision must emphasize the use of residual vision. Frequently, a low vision training assistant with a background of experience in teaching "blind" techniques will neglect training in the use of remaining vision. Different types of reinforcement are often needed to keep the patient's enthusiasm and motivation at a high level.

Enhancing the Visual Environment

It has been known for many years that the normal aging processes within the eye effectively reduce the amount of light reaching the retina. Weale (1963) states that there is on the order of a threefold drop in light transmission in a 60-year-old compared to a 20-year-old eye; that is, when exposed to the same test conditions, an average 60-year-old retina receives only one-third as much light as is received by the 20-year-old retina.

There is also increasing evidence that the contrast sensitivity of all low vision patients is reduced. In some cases, the control of the magnitude and angular distribution of the lumens flux that enter the eye can be more important than any device prescribed. Cullinan (1978) identified the importance and effects of poor lighting control for older people who were visually impaired: "Among those surveyed who have had recently been seen at a specialist's clinic, over 60% apparently saw worse at home than they did at the time of the examination." Poor lighting in the home is a prevalent problem that can dramatically inhibit the visual functioning of older people, suggesting that specification of lighting requirements for patients must be handled more effectively than it has been in the past. To meet this problem, consideration of appropriate illumination levels must include such factors as reduced light transmission levels, slower rates of adaptation to changes in lighting, and the greater likelihood of discomfort from glare. Intelligent use of lighting, color, and contrast are key aspects of the task of creating an environment in which the visually impaired person is able to make optimum use of vision.

The practitioner should be aware of potential problems with glare as light source intensities are increased. Lighting experts subdivide glare into two categories; namely discomfort glare, which is annoying and tiring but produces no measurable drop in visual acuity, and disability glare, which prevents the patient from seeing comfortably in the area of the glare source.

In setting general lighting requirements, the aim should be to remove large differences in light levels both within and between rooms. Spotlights that give a pattern of strongly highlighted and relatively shadowed areas may be striking and original to normally sighted people but totally confusing to someone with impaired vision. A more even level of illumination is preferred. It need not necessarily be of very high intensity in general living areas as long as it is supplemented by adequate lighting for the specific immediate tasks. It is important to recognize that somewhat higher illuminance levels are needed in areas that may present safety hazards such as stairs or in cooking areas.

Other Factors in Low Vision Rehabilitation

Low vision rehabilitation includes not only the prescription of appropriate low vision devices, but also instruction and supportive services to enhance the person's performance in the tasks of daily living (Rosenbloom, 1984). Adaptive training involves relearning processes that may include altering eye movements with the use of low vision devices at various fixation distances, determining the appropriate illumination for a particular task, and developing a modified procedure for the recognition of letters and words.

Various studies have reported a greater than 80 percent success rate in rehabilitating low vision patients who previously were thought to be "hopeless" (Fried, 1980; Kirchner & Phillips, 1988). Both the team approach and a professional's positive attitudes toward low vision rehabilitation are essential contributing factors.

Although elderly persons may find it difficult to compensate for vision loss through increased reliance on their other senses, the augmentation of the quality and quantity of sensory stimuli enhances their information about the environment and should facilitate their adjustments to new roles in life. For example, the use of auditory informational input, such as that provided by cassettes and Talking Books or computers with speech synthesizers, can be increased. Additional environmental information can be gained through the tactile senses; thus, the use of a cane or walker may provide a great deal of information through the sense of touch in addition to adding stability. Other sensory modalities may also be used more extensively; adaptations can be made to the environment; low vision rehabilitation involving the optometrist, ophthalmologist, and allied health care providers can be obtained; and social support systems can be used.

Low vision rehabilitation must be a team effort of all personnel who provide patient care. It is most essential that the practitioner be aware of the other resources and disciplines that relate to treating the individual as a whole person. The concept of providing optimal low vision care frequently involves the need for additional professional services; yet in this age of specialization, all too often professionals fail to look outside the narrow borders of their own disciplines because of a conscious or unconscious assumption that treatment is centered about that profession.

The overall aim in rehabilitation must be to facilitate transition from dependence to independence, and finally to interdependence. Comments typical of many patients illustrate the progression through these stages. Dependence is demonstrated by such statements as, "Of course I can't read. You'll have to do it for me." Although not as readily apparent, task avoidance is another form of dependence: "This print is just too small—no, you can't help me. I didn't want to read it anyway." Developing independence can be expressed by, "I'll try to read this myself." A typical statement of interdependence might be, "I can read this section, but those words are too difficult. Could you help me, please?" In this desirable stage of rehabilitation the individual recognizes both abilities and limitations and graciously accepts assistance. This rehabilitation process requires time, and a patient may fluctuate among these stages.

NEW DIRECTIONS IN LOW VISION CARE

The focus for the future must be in two directions—*research* and *development. Research* is the first major focus. There are a number of research directions to consider (see also Chapter 9).

There is a need for new techniques in the assessment of visual performance. As assessment procedures become more refined, there will be an improved correlation between clinical measurements of visual function and the real-world demonstration of visual skills related to a person's lifestyle. To realize this goal, research entails the creation of instrumentation capable of measuring visual functions. There is also a need for expanded research into the visual processes involved in day-to-day living.

There is a continuing challenge to design low vision devices so as to increase their application, versatility, and acceptability. In part the ophthalmic industry has responded with the production of new devices that make use of the greater design freedoms offered by new ophthalmic materials of varying indexes of refraction. More needs to be done, however.

The challenges are both technical and practical in nature. The technical challenge lies in optimizing lens design parameters. Researchers need to provide low vision corrections that combine magnification with distortion-free fields of view. There is also a practical challenge. The devices prescribed and the advice given to the low vision patient must be eminently usable.

Further research will also lead to the continued development of nonoptical aids appropriate to the level of disability and handicap. This is an area in which increased observation and innovation will bring results. This research area is particularly promising as it utilizes technological advances in other fields, such as the use of print-to-speech synthesizers.

There is also a demand for continuing research into the visual performance characteristics of the various conditions that cause loss of vision. As this research progresses, it may in turn lead to the development of new procedures for alleviating the effects of such conditions as age-related macular degeneration.

New approaches in ocular surgery offer promising future possibilities. These include the continuing development and refinement of surgical techniques in replacing nonfunctional retinal tissues in such diseases as macular degeneration and retinitis pigmentosa.

A particularly interesting area of research is the study of the process by which elderly patients relearn skills necessary for successful use of residual vision. This process of readaptation is little understood at this time. One of the challenges in the treatment of low vision is to develop suitable readaptation techniques. It would involve, for example, perceptual relearning, the use of eccentric fixation (shifting the gaze to use functional areas of the retina to avoid blind spots), and methods for expanding the functional field of vision.

A related and critically important research need is an expanded understanding of the role of the visual environment to successful readaptation. Study of lighting may involve such factors as intensity, spectral characteristics, heat properties, contrast, and the type of lighting fixtures that are most effective in various home and work environments.

The prevalence of managed care within the United States makes it essential to carry out a variety of research studies in this area. These would evaluate the impact of managed care on quality of care, patient eligibility, service delivery, and funding. Because the majority of low vision patients are over 70 years of age, the trend toward including Medicare funding within the scope of health maintenance organization (HMO) coverage underscores the significance of evaluating the effectiveness of services and quality of care.

Development as the second major focus must concentrate on the delivery of care to elderly visually impaired persons. The care of the elderly patient especially requires interdisciplinary liaison among representatives from the various professions involved. One way to achieve this liaison is the development of comprehensive multidisciplinary training centers. Such centers would be staffed by specialists in the basic clinical, social, and public health sciences. These centers would encompass not only studies of patient care delivery, but also evaluation in planning the elements comprising total low vision rehabilitation. Provisions for training of personnel and research on the effectiveness of interdisciplinary approaches would also be essential. Such centers or institutions would have responsibility for the prevention of disability by means of enhanced diagnosis, treatment, and rehabilitation of visually impaired persons.

There is also a need for in-service training to develop a highly desirable, comprehensive approach to patient care. Achieving successful rehabilitation requires close coordination among members of the rehabilitation team. This team may consist of such professionals as optometrists, ophthalmologists, social workers, occupational therapists, rehabilitation teachers, orientation and mobility (O&M) instructors, psychologists, agency administrators, low vision assistants, and many others.

Providing successful services to the low vision patient requires a service delivery system with economically viable provisions for specialized assessment, ongoing support structure, and personnel training programs. The dissemination of information about these new techniques and organizational structures is vital to the success of this process.

To evaluate the quality and efficacy of agency services, the professional team must recognize and encourage the importance of patient feedback. Without exaggeration, it is safe to say that the most important member of any team is the low vision patient himself or herself. A variety of approaches may be necessary to elicit valuable feedback.

These are the collective challenges. It is vitally important for all allied professionals to cooperate in research, apply valid research findings to improve clinical practice, and then develop practice methodologies that have a solid foundation in research. Truly, all of those professionals have a shared destiny in recommitting their best efforts to meeting these new challenges in the adventurous years that lie ahead in the new millennium.

REFERENCES

Abeles, R. P., Gift, H. C., & Ory, M. G. (1994). *Aging and quality of life.* New York: Springer.

American Association of Retired Persons & United States Administration on Aging. (1991). *A profile of older Americans.* Washington, DC.

Bortz, W. M. (1989). Redefining human aging. *Journal of the American Geriatric Society, 37,* 1092–1096.

Carter, J. H. (1982). Predictable visual responses to increasing age. *Journal of the American Optometric Association, 53,* 31–36.

Corn, A. L., & Koenig, A. J. (1996). *Foundations of low vision: Clinical and functional perspectives.* New York: AFB Press.

Cullinan, T. (1978). *Low vision in elderly people: Light for low vision.* Proceedings of a symposium, London: University College.

Cunningham, P. & Johnston, A. (1980). Edge Detection: A New Test of Visual Function. ANZAAS Jubilee Conference, Adelaide, Australia.

Freeman, P. B., & Jose, R. T. (1991). *The art and practice of low vision.* Newton, MA: Butterworth-Heinemann.

Fried, A. N. (1980). Rehabilitation: An essential component of low vision care. In Low vision ahead: Proceedings of the First Australian Pacific Conference on Low Vision, Melbourne, Australia: Australian National Council of and for the Blind, Association for the Blind.

Hiatt, L. G. (1990). Environmental factors in rehabilitation. In S. J. Brody & L. G. Pawlson, (Eds.), *Aging and rehabilitation II.* New York: Springer, pp. 151–153.

International Classification of Diseases, 9th Revision (1978). Geneva: World Health Organization.

Kanski, J. J. (1999). *Clinical ophthalmology* (4th ed.). Newton, MA: Butterworth-Heinemann.

Kirchner, C., & Phillips, B. (1988). Report of a survey of U.S. low vision services. In C. Kirchner (Ed.), *Data on blindness and visual impairment in the U.S.* (2nd ed.). New York: AFB Press, pp. 285–293.

Lubinas, J. (1980). Understanding the low vision patient. *Australian Journal of Optometry, 63* (5), 227–231.

Mehr, E. B., & Fried, A.N. (1975). *Low vision care.* Chicago: Professional Press.

Melore, G. G. (1997). Visual function changing in the geriatric patient and environmental modifications. In G. Melore (Ed), *Treating vision problems in the older adult.* St. Louis: Mosby-Yearbook, pp. 158–169.

Moore, E. J., Graves, W. H., & Patterson, J. B. (1997). *Foundations of rehabilitation counseling with persons who are blind or visually impaired.* New York: AFB Press.

Morgan, M. (1988). Vision through my aging eyes. *Journal of the American Optometric Association, 59,* 278–280.

Nelson, K. A. (1987). Statistical Briefs #35: Visual impairment among elderly Americans: Statistics in transitions. *Journal of Visual Impairment and Blindness, 80,* 331–334.

Nowakowski, R. W. (1994). *Primary low vision care.* Norwalk, CT: Appleton & Lange.

Orr, A. L. (1992). *Vision and aging: Crossroads for service delivery.* New York: AFB Press.

Recommended practice for lighting and the visual environment for senior living. (1998). Prepared by the IESNA Lighting and Partially Sighted Committee. New York: Illuminating Engineering Society of North America.

Rosenbloom, A. (1984). An Overview of Low Vision Care: Accomplishments and Ongoing Problems, *Journal of Visual Impairment & Blindness, 78,* 491–493.

Rosenbloom, A., & Morgan, M. (1993). *Vision and aging* (2nd ed.). Stoneham, MA: Butterworth-Heinemann.

Rubin, G. S., West, S. K., Munoz, B., Bardeen-Roche, K., Zegere, S., Achein, O., & Fried, L. P. (1997). A comprehensive assessment of visual impairment in a population of older American, The SEE Study, Salisbury Eye Evaluation Project. *Investigative Ophthalmalogy and Visual Science, 38,* 557–568.

Sekuler, R., Kline, D., & Dismukes, K. (1982). *Aging and human visual function.* New York: Alan R. Liss.

Tielsch, J. M., Sommer, A., Witt, K., Katz, J., & Royall, R. M. (1990). Blindness and visual impairment in an American urban population, The Baltimore Eye Survey. *Archives of Ophthalmology, 108,* 286–290.

Vaughn, D., Asbury, T., & Riordan-Eva, P. (1995). *General Ophthalmology* (14th ed.). Norwalk, CT: Appleton & Lange.

Vision problems in the United States: Facts and figures (1980). New York: National Society to Prevent Blindness.

Weale, R. A. (1963). *The aging eye.* London: H. K. Lewis & Co.

World Health Organization (1981). The use of residual vision by visually disabled persons: Report of a World Health Organization meeting. *Euro Reports and Studies No. 41,* Geneva, Switzerland: Author.

CHAPTER 5

Medical Considerations in the Rehabilitation of Older Persons

Dale C. Strasser

It is hard to imagine this chapter, or for that matter this book, being written 60 years ago. At the start of the 21st century, the challenges confronting medical and rehabilitation personnel arise from the successes that have been achieved. The last two-thirds of the 20th century have witnessed incredible advances in health care. From improvements in sanitation and public health to the advent of antibiotics and the successes of whole organ transplants, today health care practitioners and their patients are presented with an impressive and bewildering spectrum of options. In conjunction with significant improvements in sanitation, nutrition, and public health, humans are enjoying longer and healthier lives than ever before.

Although growing old is not easy, it is important to remember that the possibility of large numbers of adults living to such ages simply did not exist in the past. At present, the majority of older adults in the United States enjoy generally good health and are community-dwelling productive citizens without evidence of dementia. Not only can older adults learn new skills, but some intellectual skills (such as those based on procedural knowledge) continue to improve well into the seventh decade of life. A recent book sponsored by the MacArthur

Foundation, *Successful Aging* (Rowe & Kahn, 1998), compiles an impressive summary of scientific findings to dispel negative stereotypes and myths about aging.

So why do these myths persist? In part these sentiments exist because there are elements of truth embedded within them. The usual life course in industrialized countries ends in death in the eighth to ninth decade, and commonly death is preceded by a period of increasing functional limitations. The reality of functional decline taps into basic human fears of loss and mortality. Not only do older adults experience a generalized loss of functional capacity as part of biological ("normal") aging, but the incidence of most disabling medical diseases (e.g., stroke and dementia) also increases with age. The underlying decline in functional capacity associated with the biology of aging may remain dormant for extended periods. However, with the diminished functional reserves associated with aging, the effects of physical impairments such as vision loss tend to be more pronounced for older than for younger individuals.

The ageist myths challenged by Rowe and Kahn (1998) exist because we have the luxury of contemplating our own mortality over a prolonged period of time, and that experience can be disconcerting. There is an understandable subtext in health care and rehabilitation to view the problems of contemporary society as ones of enormous gravity with bleak overtones. It is important to keep in mind, however, that the current circumstances have resulted from tremendous successes.

Vision loss in later life adds a distinct complexity to the challenges of successful aging. As individuals grow older, they typically experience a gradual decline in functional reserves and, later on, functional capacities. Between ages 20 and 50, most people begin to notice a loss in capabilities such as physical endurance, high-frequency hearing, rote memory, and night vision, but they learn to accommodate. The good news is that effective rehabilitation strategies are available to facilitate adaptation, which contribute to the effectiveness of the increasing number of medical and surgical options.

As reviewed in Chapter 2, demographic changes in modern society are mind boggling. With the combination of increasing life expectancy and decreasing birth rate, industrialized societies in particular are undergoing enormous demographic changes. Whereas approximately 4 percent of the U.S. population was 65 years old or older at the turn of the century, this number had grown to 13 percent, or 33 million, by 1994 (Cohen & Van Nostrand, 1995). In contrast, the higher birth rates and hence lower average age in developing countries mask the fact that worldwide a majority of older adults live in developing countries and that this numerical majority is increasing (U.S. Bureau of the Census, 1992).

This chapter places aging and vision rehabilitation in the context of medicine and medical rehabilitation. It begins with a historical perspective on why rehabilitation in the field of blindness and low vision has been mostly neglected in the medical specialty of physical medicine and rehabilitation. Then, a short review of the biology of aging is offered as a foundation for a statement of salient principles in geriatric medicine. The construct of frailty as decreased reserves—which may be biological, psychological, or social—is discussed as a framework to understand the intertwined roles of medicine and rehabilitation in assisting older adults to achieve their optimal functional capabilities. The chapter concludes with suggestions on devising effective rehabilitation interventions for older adults with visual impairments.

MEDICAL REHABILITATION AND SERVICES FOR INDIVIDUALS WHO ARE BLIND OR VISUALLY IMPAIRED

In the United States, medical rehabilitation underwent tremendous growth during World War II. Faced with large numbers of disabled veterans, pioneers such as the internist Howard Rusk (1977) developed multidisciplinary strategies to enable injured soldiers to return to productive life. The principles of medical rehabilitation in the United States arose to a large extent from these rehabilitative strategies developed during World War II.

Initially, activities within medical rehabilitation were closely aligned with vocational rehabilitation (Kottke & Knapp, 1988; Rusk, 1977). The field of vocational rehabilitation was able to provide models of functional restoration, adaptive equipment, and compensatory strategies utilizing multidisciplinary teams, not to mention an established bureaucracy with political clout. Understandably, the occurrence of war-related injuries presented some distinct issues in comparison to the prewar situation, including an increase in acute medical problems and a preponderance of orthopedic and neurological injuries.

Although it continued to be aligned with vocational rehabilitation, medical rehabilitation in the 1940s evolved into a medical specialty. This medical orientation was attributable, in part, to the acute medical needs of the patients. Furthermore, the incorporation of rehabilitation (of some conditions) into medicine added a credibility to rehabilitation and increased options for funding sources (Kottke & Knapp, 1988). As this evolution continued, some areas, such as blind rehabilitation, tended to stay within vocational rehabilitation, whereas other areas, such as acute injuries (e.g., spinal cord and traumatic brain injury) and stroke, fell under the purview of rehabilitation medicine. The relative importance of "vocational" issues gradually receded as the post–World War II population aged and an increasing number of individuals with disabilities were near or past retirement age. This curious set of influences resulted in a partial separation of rehabilitation services for visual impairments from services for physical and cognitive disabilities.

REHABILITATION AND GERIATRIC MEDICINE

In the United States and the United Kingdom, the medical areas of rehabilitation and geriatrics show interesting similarities and contrasts (Strasser, 1992). In the 1930s, Dr. Marjory Warren in the United Kingdom spearheaded efforts to address the medical and functional needs of a predominately older patient group in a large London hospital dedicated to the care of chronic conditions (Matthews & Warren, 1984). She developed what is now referred to as a comprehensive geriatric assessment, involving a multidisciplinary team that concentrated on the improvement of physical functional abilities. Her remarkable efforts resulted in the transfer of nearly 80 percent of the "incurables" to the community. Her team developed compensatory strategies and assistive devices such as canes and sliding boards (referred to as "shuffle boards") to enhance independence of transfers into and out of bed. Dr. Warren's work laid the foundation for geriatric medicine—initially in the United Kingdom and later in the United States.

With no apparent awareness of Warren's work, Dr. Howard Rusk pioneered medical rehabilitation efforts in the United States while caring for soldiers injured in World War II. Rusk devised strategies to rehabilitate this younger and acutely disabled group. During the process, he championed the importance of functional evaluation and multidisiciplinary interventions. In his autobiography, Rusk (1977) documents the obstacles he encountered in instituting therapeutic exercise programs. The medical profession at the time did not appreciate the value of reconditioning: an illness was followed by convalescence, and then the individual was "well."

The similar approaches developed for these two different population groups suggest some universal principles for the management of people with disabilities (Strasser, 1992). Effective interventions are practical, comprehensive, and multidisciplinary. Biopsychosocial concerns should be addressed to achieve optimal results. It is also noteworthy that these two pioneers of geriatrics and rehabilitation rarely addressed specifically the needs of people with visual impairments. Both emphasized the orthopedic, neurological, and generalized deconditioning issues of their patients.

BIOLOGY OF AGING

It is generally accepted that as individuals age a series of genetically determined biological changes unfold. From infancy to old age, these parameters set the stage for the individual's capability for human activities. Intertwined with normal biological aging, however, are a host of mitigating factors, including the social and physical environments, cultural variables, and disease. Although it can be very difficult to untangle these influences in a given circumstance, there has been a tremendous increase in the basic understanding of the biology of aging over the past several decades. (For more detailed reviews of the biology of aging and rehabilitation, see Alonzo and Cote [1994] and Clark & Siebens [1998]).

Physiological Systems

As individuals grow older, the performance of the cardiovascular system declines, showing an increasing "stiffness" within the system and altered electrical conduction within the heart. At the cellular level, the stiffness or decreased compliance (the ability to expand) within the cardiovascular system is associated with increased amounts of lipofuscin, connective tissue, and lipid deposits. Concurrent with these changes, the left ventrical of the heart enlarges, and resting heart rate, blood pressure, and norepinephrine (or adrenaline) levels increase. These changes occur simultaneously with increases in blood pressure and decreases in maximum heart rate, VO_2 max (an accepted measure of cardiac capabilities), and orthostatic blood pressure responses, changes that are all associated with aging. These effects help explain the overall decline in cardiovascular fitness associated with aging. As documented by Rowe and Kahn (1998), numerous studies have shown that many of the changes can be modified significantly through regular physical exercise.

Similar themes characterize age-associated change in the pulmonary systems as well. The changes in pulmonary functions as individuals age follow logically from the observed diminished compliance both within the chest wall and in the elastic recoil of the lung. Furthermore, there are age-associated decreases in the efficiency of gas (e.g., oxygen–carbon dioxide) exchange. Clinically these changes are observed as increases in functional residual capacity (FRC) and residual volume (RV) and decreases in vital capacity (VC). In brief, the pulmonicial system becomes stiffer and less capable of withstanding physiological stress. The effects of these changes increase the work of breathing.

Medical rehabilitation professionals take particular interest in age-associated changes in the muscular system. These include muscle atrophy and a decrease in muscle strength, even though relative muscular endurance may not be affected by age. The age-associated decrease in muscle strength is associated with both a reduction in the number of functional motor units and a tendency for lower levels of physical activty. Of the two primary muscle fiber types (Type I or "fast twitch" and Type II or "slow twitch"), a relative atrophy in Type II muscle fibers has been associated with age (Larsson and Karlsson, 1978). These "fast-twitch" fibers are capable of generating large forces quickly, and hence their atrophy corresponds to the observed decrease in muscle strength. Type I muscle fibers ("slow-twitch") are better suited for less intense effort over a longer time. The relative preservation of Type I over Type II muscle fibers helps explain the maintenance of muscle endurance with age.

Vision changes are some of the most commonly recognized age-associated changes. Presbyopia is experienced by the overwhelming number of adults over the age of 65. This loss of the ability to focus on near objects results from a deterioriation in the ability to increase the thickness and curvature of the lens. Likewise, a decrease in tolerance of glare and formation of cataracts occur to some degree in most older adults. In addition to these usual vision changes with aging, older individuals are at higher risk for eye diseases including glaucoma, macular degeneration, and diabetic retinopathy. (For a more detailed discussion of age-associated visual changes and disease conditions, see Chapter 4.)

Similar themes are pervasive in other body systems as well. For example, in the skeletal system, older people experience loss of bone mass (osteoporosis) and tissue flexibility. In the renal system, kidneys lose mass, and there is a decrement in filtration rate. Red blood cells and other elements of the hematopoietic (formation of blood cells) system are slower to recover from physiological insult. Glucose tolerance decreases, increasing the risk of diabetes.

Generally speaking, studies in the biology of aging reveal a gradual loss of physiological capacities. These changes may not have any functional implications for the individual, however. The same individual at ages 20, 50, or 80 may not experience any functional decline in most or all major physiological systems. Typically, however, there is a loss of functional reserve over an individual's life span, experienced as an inability to recover from physiological stress. A urinary tract infection, for example, may be an annoyance to a 40-year-old; the same infection may have profound ramifications on an 80-year-old's ability to live independently in the community. For the latter individual, the infection may initiate a cascade of events, such as adverse reactions to medication, delirium, dehydration, and injurious falls, which compromise the older person's ability to continue living safely in the community.

Neurological Function

Age-associated changes in the nervous system are of particular importance for rehabilitation professions, because the status of the nervous system influences the ability to successfully implement the compensatory strategies that underlie many rehabilitation interventions (Chancellor & Borkow, 1994). Although the ability to retain a large body of information declines, general intelligence in the absence of disease is well maintained into a person's 80s. Other neurological functions show decline with age. A few examples reveal the potential influence of neurological changes on rehabilitation. Postural reflexes and balance reactions tend to be slower in older adults. It follows that an older adult with visual impairment is at increased risk for injuries such as hip fractures as a result of falls (Cooper & Barker, 1995).

Illness

Commonly it is a medical illness, rather than the age-associated biological changes, that may affect functional abilities that tips the scale from simply decreased functional reserves to true functional disabilities. Furthermore, most chronic medical conditions, such as heart disease, stroke, diabetes, Alzheimer's disease, and Parkinson's disease, tend to increase in frequency with age. It is rare that an older individual with a visual impairment does not have at least one or more chronic diseases. In turn, these chronic conditions become risk factors for disabling conditions. For example, not only does the probability of an older adult experiencing a hip fracture increase with the presence of particular risk factors, but the relationship is more synergistic than additive (Cooper & Barker, 1995; Zuckerman, 1996). With the exception of early childhood, the likelihood of an individual experiencing serious medical conditions and decreasing physiological reserves increases with age.

BIOPSYCHOSOCIAL DIMENSIONS OF FRAILTY

Frailty provides a useful construct for understanding the functional disabilities of disabled older adults (Buckner & Wagner, 1992). Many professionals find it useful to expand the construct of frailty beyond physiological parameters to include psychological, social, and economic concerns. Frailty may be thought of as the limited reserves an individual has in his or her global functioning. These limited reserves can occur in one or more of the many domains influencing an individual's ability to function. Frailty can be thought of as the inverse of stress tolerance. Frail individuals have diminished functional reserves and are more likely to become disabled under stress. This stress may have predominately social, psychological, or physical origins, or more commonly, it may be a product of limitations in multiple domains. As shown in Figure 1, an individual's success in withstanding stress in a given environment is a function of age-associated changes, age-related medical conditions, and psychosocial factors.

Frailty does not equate with illness, disease, or activity limitation, but rather it increases the possibilities for these and related conditions to become manifest under particular circumstances. A more robust individual is more likely to withstand stress successfully than someone who is frail. Disability increases frailty, that is, decreases reserves. Individuals who are disabled are, by this definition, frail (e.g., at increased risk), even though frail individuals are not necessarily disabled.

A relationship can be proposed between the recently updated World Health Organization's (WHO) *International Classification of Functioning and Disability,* ICIDH-2 (World Health Organization, 1999), and this construct of frailty in Figure 2. In WHO's schema, a particular disease leads to altered physiological function, or impairment; activity limitation (previously referred to as disability) is

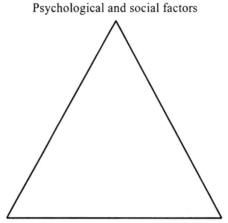

Psychological and social factors

Age-related medical conditions   Age-associated changes

Figure 1
Success in Withstanding Stress as a Function of Age-associated Changes, Age-related Medical Conditions, and Psychosocial Factors

the extent to which an individual is unable to perform basic activities of daily living, and participation or participation restriction (previously referred to as handicap) reflects the degree of change in social role bought about by the disease.[1] When a construct of frailty is added to the WHO schema, frailty can be viewed in biological, psychological, and social dimensions. Frailty increases the risks of impairment, activity limitation, and participation restriction. The body, the individual, and social realms are offered as intermediary steps relating frailty with the WHO classification. In the proposed combination of frailty and the WHO schema, the effects of biological aging and disease are initially seen in bodily functions and hence relate to impairment. The diminished reserves or frailty of an individual in performing basic activities of daily living is manifest at the level of the individual as activity limitation; frailty in performing one's social role at the level of the community manifests itself as participation

---

[1]Some readers may prefer the Institute of Medicine (IOM) model of "disablement" (Brandt & Pope, 1997). Although subtleties exist between the WHO and IOM models, for our purposes the IOM's constructs of impairment, functional limitation, and disability closely parallel the WHO's constructs of impairment, activity limitation, and participation.

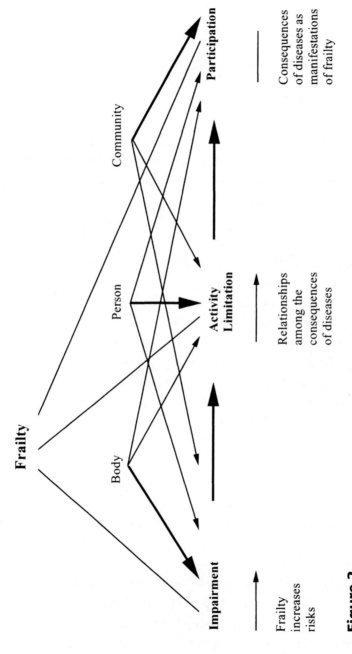

Figure 2
Frailty and the World Health Organization's Schema of the Effects of Disease

restriction. The constructs of frailty and functional abilities have interrelated influences derived from the myriad of biopsychosocial influences.

REHABILITATION AND EXERCISE

Frail elderly individuals with disabilities do show improvements with rehabilitation. In medical rehabilitation, the role of exercise appears to be one of the building blocks of successful interventions. Perhaps no topic in geriatrics and rehabilitation has been so thoroughly studied and shown to be as beneficial as exercise. Sedentary older adults show benefit in most of the age-associated changes described above including cardiovascular parameters, muscle activity (strength and aerobic enzyme activity), increase in bone mass, improved glucose tolerance, and even cognitive alertness (Buckner et al., 1997; Fiatarone, Marks, Ryan, Meredith, Lipsitz, & Evans, 1990).

Generally speaking, increased activity and exercise are good for young and old people alike. Occasionally, medical conditions exist in which the ongoing participation or supervision by medical personnel is indicated. These include cardiovascular (e.g., coronary artery disease, arrhythmias, and peripheral vascular disease), neuromuscular (e.g., muscle and motor neuron diseases, post-polio syndrome), and others (e.g., diabetes). Medical consultation is recommended for older adults when establishing activity parameters and an exercise program.

More commonly the challenge to implementing an effective exercise program is the compliance of the individual. Researchers at the Atlanta VA Rehabilitation Research and Development Center (Boyette & Boyette, 1998) are spearheading an expert system that attempts to meld the insights of a proper exercise prescription with maximum client compliance into a computer software program. Perhaps enjoyment and convenience are the most important factors in maintaining an exercise program. Other factors include congruence with the patient's lifestyle, opportunity for social interaction, program cost, and level of physical discomfort.

In more physiological terms, exercise prescriptions typically factor in endurance, strength, and flexibility concerns. Target heart rates, such as 65 percent to 75 percent of maximum, and exercise duration are specified in the endurance and aerobic-conditioning goals of an exercise prescription. Warm-up and cool-down portions of an exercise program typically consist of low-intensity stretching and range-of-motion activities. These activities help prepare the body for more strenuous activity and reduce the risk of injury and exercise-induced arrhythmias. Weight-lifting is a form of strength training. The study of Fiatarone et al. (1990) among elderly cognitively impaired nursing home residents showed beneficial results from a strength training program. Clinical experience suggests relatively high compliance for walking and swimming activities. Recent work on T'ai Chi with older adults has found impressive rates of compliance. Functional benefits include reduction in the risks of injurious falls (Wolf et al., 1996).

In addition to the general health benefits of an exercise program, recent studies have confirmed the benefits of medical rehabilitation for frail, older adults even though earlier studies did not find such benefits (Jette, Harris, Cleary, & Campion, 1987; Schuman, Beattie, Steed, Merry, & Kraus, 1981). Clinical experience suggests that well-designed rehabilitation interventions can promote the achievement of meaningful goals and help older adults who have disabling conditions to remain in the community. Important factors in achieving optimal outcomes appear to include a realistic assessment of the patient's current status and functional potential. This assessment should include an individual's biological, psychological, and social circumstances. Are the rehabilitation goals congruent with the patient's goals? Is there a reasonable chance that the proposed intervention will make a difference? Medical rehabilitation professionals have a spectrum of rehabilitation venues to consider for a disabled older adult, such as rehabilitation provided in the acute, the subacute, outpatient, or home settings. Unfortunately, health care provider convenience, financial considerations (the patient's, practitioner's, and institution's), and the current trend to allow only short lengths of hospital stays for acute conditions exert a significant influence on an individual as a rehabilitation candidate and where the services should be provided.

SYNDROMES IN GERIATRIC MEDICINE

Distinctive characteristics of geriatric medicine, in contrast to acute care medicine, can be seen in the identification of common syndromes in geriatrics. Typically, older adults seeking medical attention have not one but multiple underlying medical conditions. The list of medical problems grows as one ages. Common entities on this list may include diabetes, cataracts, hypertension, atrial fibrillation, and coronary artery disease. As geriatricians strive to manage these issues in an optimal manner, the distinctive contribution of geriatric medicine is to incorporate these discrete medical conditions into a patient- and family-centered and functionally oriented approach to medical assessment and intervention plans. From this orientation geriatricians, gerontologists, and other health care specialists have developed assessment and intervention strategies that address these functional concerns.

Common syndromes highlighted in geriatric medicine include the so-called "3 Ds" (dementia, depression, delirium), falls and fractures, and urinary incontinence. These syndromes capture functionally significant issues that medical personnel encounter in older patients. Furthermore, health professionals experienced in the field of aging discovered that older adults were particularly susceptible to iatrogenic illnesses. Polypharmacy, or the inappropriate use of medications resulting in undesirable and potentially grave side effects, was identified as a major source of physician-induced medical problems, along with inappropriate tests and medical interventions. Inadequate intervention was also of concern and included limited attention to functional abilities, to ameliorating age-associated biological changes and disease, to optimizing caregiver involvement, and to death and dying. Hence enlightened health professionals, particularly geriatricians and gerontologists, are refocusing health care toward a more geriatric-friendly approach. Although it seems somewhat trite, health care professionals cannot cure death, but they can enhance the quality of life.

Difficulties with cognition and affect are a major theme in promoting optimal functioning in older adults. Even though only 10 percent of the U.S. population age 65 years and older shows evidence of Alzheimer's disease, the incidence of this disease increases exponentially after the age of 65. Although only 5 percent of those between 65 and 74 years of age showed evidence of Alzheimer's in one large community-based study, the incidence increased to nearly 20 percent in the 75- to 84-year-old group, and nearly 50 percent in those 85 and older (Brookmeyer, Gray, & Kawas, 1998). Although other studies have found somewhat different rates (summarized in Alonzo & Cote, 1994; Poon, 1985), the theme of dramatic increases in the incidence of Alzheimer's disease with age remains consistent. Combined with the fact that the oldest-old (those aged 85 and older) is the fastest growing demographic group in the United States, rehabilitation professionals must continue to develop strategies to deal with multiple chronic conditions simultaneously.

Hip fractures comprise one of the most common sources of disability in the elderly population, and visual impairment is a risk factor for sustaining a hip fracture. The extent to which cognitively impaired older adults suffering from a hip fracture benefit from rehabilitation remains controversial. Several studies (Jette et al., 1987; Schuman, Beattie, Steed, Merry, & Kraus, 1981) failed to show that these patients made significant gains with intensive rehabilitation. Clinical experience and more recent work (Goldstein, Strasser, Woodward, & Roberts, 1997) suggest that these individuals can make significant improvements in rehabilitation programs tailored to their needs. The success of some rehabilitation efforts but not others may reflect the nature of the intervention itself. Rehabilitation is not one prescribed intervention, but an approach to teaching new skills. Some professionals believe that there may be an inadvertent age bias among medical rehabilitation providers that may influence their effectiveness (Hesse, Campion, & Karamouz, 1984). Such beliefs have been supported by studies on staff attitudes (Kvitek, Shaver, Blood, & Shepard, 1986; Strasser, Falconer, & Martino-Saltzmann, 1992) and the distinctive characteristics of older adults in rehabilitation settings (Falconer, Naughton, Strasser, & Sinacore, 1994).

Insights into the apparent discrepancies in the effectiveness of rehabilitation treatment across settings may reflect the compatibility between the treatment environment and the elderly, demented patient's learning styles. Studies on learning and cognitive impairments in diverse conditions, such as traumatic brain injury and Alzheimer's disease (Ewert, Levin, Watson, & Kalisky, 1989), have uncovered similar themes. Cognitive impairment does not affect all types of learning in the same way. Procedural learning, which involves the motor action itself, is more resilient to cognitive insult than declarative learning, which is primarily language based. Hence, overlearned motor skills, such as walking and toileting, appear to be more amenable to relearning than new language-based skills for individuals with cognitive impairment. Some of the success of rehabilitation efforts may be based on the success of these interventions to tap into procedural as opposed to declarative learning strategies.

In contrast to dementia, delirium is characterized as reversible alteration in consciousness of limited duration. Nearly everyone has experienced a degree of delirium. Common precipitating causes include alcohol consumption, sleep deprivation, pain medication, and excessive environmental stimulation. This author has experienced a degree of delirium shopping in crowded malls during the holiday season in conjunction with low blood sugar! The risk of delirium increases with increased number of risk factors (e.g., medications, dementia, psychological stress, and unfamiliar environment). The general approach to delirium is to treat underlying medical and environmental conditions and to reduce risk factors.

Late-onset depression commonly contributes to functional decline in older adults (Katz & Alexopoulos, 1996). This variant of depression has aspects in common with depression affecting some individuals in middle age (e.g., changes in affect, appetite, and patterns of sleep and physical activity) as well as some distinctive characteristics (e.g., pseudodementia, somatic complaints, and gastrointestinal disturbances). In addition to these signs and symptoms of late-onset depression, clinical experience suggests that anhedonia, or the lack of pleasure in most if not all activities, is helpful in diagnosing depression. In the last 20 years, tremendous strides have been achieved in medical management of late onset depression. In conjunction with improved understanding of the physiological and environmental contributions to depression (see review articles in Katz & Alexopoulos, 1996), effective interventions with improved side-effect profiles have been developed including psychopharmacology and electroconvulsive therapy. These medical interventions enhance the positive contributions of counseling, psychotherapy, and environmental modifications. Furthermore, clinical experience and common sense suggest that meaningful improvements in physical functioning elevate mood.

In assessing functionally impaired older adults, untangling the relative contributions of dementia, delirium, and depression is paramount to devising the most effective geriatric rehabilitation intervention. Each of the "3 Ds" can interact with the others to aggravate functional decline. There are strategies that enhance the management of dementia (Mace & Rabins, 1991). Recent advances in medical treatment of Alzheimer's disease, including anticholinesterase medications, have been promising in slowing down the progression of the disease. Clearly, progress has been made in the past two decades in the assessment and effective intervention for depression and delirium.

Disorders of balance and injuries from falls are also another major contributing factor to functional decline in older adults. Older adults in the United States experience more than 250,000 hip fractures annually, and this is expected to double by the year 2040 (Cummings, Kelsey, Nevitt, & O'Dowd, 1985). As reviewed by Zuckerman (1996), risk factors for injurious falls include impairments in cognition, vision, balance, medications, depression, osteoporosis, and the physical environment. Older adults can have a predisposition to many of these risk factors because of age-associated biological changes. Reductions in injurious falls have been achieved through comprehensive efforts at reducing risk factors in community-dwelling older adults (Tinetti et al., 1994), in nursing homes (Ray et al., 1997), and through T'ai Chi (Wolf et al., 1996).

As amply documented in a comprehensive review (Fantl et al., 1996), urinary incontinence is a problem of enormous magnitude for older adults. In the United States alone, it is estimated that urinary incontinence affects approximately 13 million individuals at an annual cost of more than $15 billion, as well as enormous psychosocial costs for individuals, their families and caregivers, and society at large, resulting in loss of self-esteem and functional independence. Urinary incontinence is associated with poorer outcomes in rehabilitation settings (Falconer, Naughton, Dunlop, Roth, Strasser, & Sinacore, 1994; Granger, Hamilton, & Fiedler, 1992). Effective and complementary interventions using medical, nursing, behavioral, and environmental strategies have cured or improved urinary incontinence in frail elderly adults (Fantl et al., 1996; Ouslander & Schnelle, 1995).

DEVISING EFFECTIVE REHABILITATION STRATEGIES

Insights from geriatrics and rehabilitation medicine provide a helpful foundation in devising effective rehabilitation strategies for older adults with visual impairment. Rarely does visual impairment occur in the absence of other age-associated conditions. Appropriate functional assessment and medical management based on established principles of geriatric medicine are critical to setting the stage for effective rehabilitation interventions. Functional assessment and medical management inevitably involve a multidisciplinary approach. The interventions should be coordinated and integrated into a cohesive framework. Studies support the clinical suspicion that frail, disabled older adults have better outcomes from coordinated care than from medical interventions that are not specifically coordinated (Applegate et al., 1990; Rubenstein et al., 1984).

Anecdotal and empirical evidence in fact suggests that rehabilitation professionals may be insensitive to the needs of older individuals (Strasser, 1992). Two contributing factors are proposed. Older adults with visual impairments tend to have multiple medical problems and hence multiple contributions to their functional disabilities. Rehabilitation professionals who prefer straightforward cases whereby a patient's disability occurs exclusively in the professional's area of expertise will probably become frustrated with complex and interrelated factors contributing to an elderly person's disability. Another stumbling block for designing effective rehabilitation strategies for this group arises from poor appreciation of age-associated changes in cognition and learning (Kvitek et al., 1984). Learning styles differ in learners in their early 20s and in those over the age of 60 (Chancellor & Borkow, 1994; Rentz, 1991). Younger learners are more likely to take risks; older learners tend to be more risk averse. The personal goals and effective reinforcements may differ between young people and old people. Perhaps these factors contribute to observations by geriatricians and rehabilitation professionals that the medical rehabilitation environment is more geared to younger people with disabilities than to older people with disabilities (Strasser, 1992).

Experience in geriatric rehabilitation suggests the following guidelines for devising effective interventions with older people who are experiencing vision loss:

- ◆ Involve the patient and caregivers in setting goals.
- ◆ Direct efforts toward meaningful functional improvement.
- ◆ Obtain the participation of medical professionals acquainted with rehabilitation strategies for individuals with impaired vision.
- ◆ Customize interventions to the physical and cognitive abilities of the patient.
- ◆ Ensure that the client perceives rehabilitation plans as relevant and fun!
- ◆ Reduce risk factors for common geriatric syndromes.

CONCLUSION

Until recently there has been a curious separation of geriatrics and medical rehabilitation on the one hand, and low vision and medical rehabilitation on the other. Medical professionals have been slow to address the functional disabilities of people with visual impairments. Correspondingly, rehabilitation efforts in the field of blindness and visual impairment may exhibit some of the same insensitivity to aging as the medical rehabilitation specialty. This chapter offers the construct of frailty as decreased functional reserves as a framework for assessment and intervention. A relatively small physiological change can have an enormous impact on the functional capabilities of a frail, elderly individual. Similarly, modest improvements in functional capabilities may have a very significant impact on the functional capabilities and living status of a frail, elderly individual. Rehabilitation assessments should build from a comprehensive biopsychosocial understanding of a patient's disability. Interventions should focus on obtainable and meaningful goals that will improve an individual's functional abilities and quality of life. Efforts, including this book, are needed to span these worlds of rehabilitation and aging.

REFERENCES

Alonzo, J. A., & Cote, L. J. (1994). Biology of aging in humans. In J. A. Downey, S. J. Myers, E. G. Gonzales, & J. S. Lieberman (Eds.), *The physiological basis of rehabilitation medicine* (2nd ed.). Boston: Butterworth-Heinemann, pp. 689–704.

Applegate, W. B., Miller, S. T., Graney, M. J., Elam, J. T., Burns, R., & Atkins, D. E. (1990). A randomized, controlled trial of a geriatric assessment unit in a community rehabilitation hospital. *New England Journal of Medicine, 322,* 1572–1578.

Boyette, L., & Boyette, J. E. (1998). Exercise program designs for older adults. *Rehabilitation R&D Progress Reports,* Department of Veterans Affairs, 103–104.

Brandt, E. N., Jr., & Pope, A. M. (Eds). (1997). *Enabling America: Assessing the role of rehabilitation science and engineering.* Washington, DC: National Academy Press.

Brookmeyer, R., Gray, S., & Kawas, C. (1998). Projections of Alzheimer's disease in the United States and the public health impact of delaying onset. *American Journal of Public Health, 88,* 1337–1341.

Buckner, D. M., & Wagner, E. H. (1992). Preventing frail health. *Clinics in Geriatric Medicine, 8(1),* 1–17.

Buckner, D. M., Cress, M. E., de Lateur, B. J., Esselman, P. C., Margherita, A. J., Price, R., & Wagner, E. H. (1997). The effect of strength and endurance training on gait, balance, fall risk, and health services use in community-living older adults. *Journal of Gerontology, 52A(4),* M218-M224.

Chancellor, Y. B., & Borkow, R. B. (1994). Central nervous system plasticity and cognitive remediation. In J. A. Downey, S. J. Myers, E. G. Gonzales, & J. S. Lieberman (Eds.), *The physiological basis of rehabilitation medicine* (2nd ed.). Boston, Butterworth-Heinemann, pp 599–624.

Clark, G. S., & Siebens, H. C. (1998). Geriatric rehabilitation. In J. A. DeLisa & B. M. Gans (Eds.), *Rehabilitation medicine: Principles and practice* (3rd ed.). Philadelphia: Lippincott-Raven, pp. 963–995.

Cohen, R. A., & Van Nostrand, J. F. (1995). Trends in the health of older Americans: United States, 1994. National Center for Health Statistics. *Vital Health Statistics 3(30)*.

Cooper, C., & Barker, D. J. P. (1995). Risk factors for hip fracture. *New England Journal of Medicine, 332(12)*, 814–815.

Cummings, S. R., Kelsey, J. L., Nevitt, M. C., O'Dowd, K. J. (1985). Epidemiology of osteoporosis and osteoporotic fractures. *Epidemiologic Reviews, 7*, 178–208.

Cummings, S. R., Phillips, S. L., Wheat, M. E., Black D., Goosby E., Wlodarczyk D., Tafton P., Jergesen H., Winograd C. H., & Hulle, S. B. (1988). Recovery of function after hip fracture: The role of social supports. *Journal of the American Geriatrics Society, 36*, 801–806.

Ewert, J., Levin, H. S., Watson, M. G., & Kalisky, Z. (1989). Procedural memory during posttraumatic amnesia in survivors of severe closed injury: Implications for rehabilitation. *Archives of Neurology, 46*, 911–916.

Falconer, J. A., Naughton, B. J., Dunlop, D. D., Roth, E. J., Strasser, D. C., & Sinacore, J. M. (1994). Predicting stroke inpatient rehabilitation outcome using a classification tree approach. *Archives of Physical Medicine and Rehabilitation, 75* 619–625.

Falconer, J. A., Naughton, B. J., Strasser, D. C., & Sinacore, J. M. (1994). Storke inpatient rehabilitation: A comparison across age groups. *Journal of the American Geriatrics Society, 42*, 39–44.

Fantl, J. A., Newman, D. K., Colling, J., Delancey, J., Norton, P., Keeyes, C., Loughly, R., McDowell, J., Ouslander, J., Schnelle, J., Staskin, D., Tries, J., Urich, V., Vitousck, S. H., Weiss, B. D., & Whitmore, K. (1996). Urinary incontinence in adults: Acute and chronic management. *Clinical Practice Guideline*, No. 2, 1996 Update. Rockville, MD: U.S. Department of Health and Human Services. Public Health Service, Agency for Health Care Policy and Research. AHCPR Publication No. 96-0682.

Fiatarone, M. A., Marks, E. C., Ryan, N.D., Meredith, C. N., Lipsitz, L. A., & Evans, W. J. (1990). High-intensity strength training in nonagenarians. *Journal of the American Medical Association, 263*, 3029.

Goldstein, F. C., Strasser, D. C., Woodward, J. L. & Roberts, V. J. (1997). Functional outcome of cognitively impaired hip fracture patients on a geriatric rehabilitation unit. *Journal of the American Geriatrics Society, 45*, 35–42.

Granger, C. V., Hamilton, B. B., & Fiedler, R. (1992).Discharge outcome after stroke rehabilitation. *Stroke, 23*, 978–982.

Hesse, K. A., Campion, E. W., & Karamouz, N. (1984). Attitudinal stumbling blocks to geriatric rehabilitation. *Journal of the American Geriatrics Society, 32*, 747–750.

Jette, A. M., Harris, B. A., Cleary, P. Campion, E. W. (1987). Functional recovery after hip fracture. *Archives of Physical Medicine and Rehabilitation, 68,* 735–740.

Katz, I. R., & Alexopoulos, G. S. (1996). Proceedings of the Geriatric Psychiatry Alliance, January 20, 1996. *The American Journal of Geriatric Psychiatry, 4(4), Suppl. 1.* Washington, D.C.: American Psychiatric Press.

Kottke, F. J., & Knapp, M. E. (1988). The development of physiatry before 1950. *Archives of Physical Medicine and Rehabilitation, 69,* 4–14.

Kvitek, S. D. B., Shaver, B. J., Blood, H., & Shepard, K. F. (1986). Age bias: Physical therapists and older patients. *Journal of Gerontology, 41,* 706–709.

Larsson, L., & Karlsson, J. (1978). Isometric and dynamic endurance as a function of age and skeletal muscle characteristics. *Acta Physiologica Scandinavica, 104,* 129–136.

Mace, N. L., & Rabins, P. V. (1991). *The 36-hour day* (revised edition), Baltimore: The Johns Hopkins University Press.

Matthews, D. A., & Warren, M. (1984). The origins of British geriatrics. *Journal of the American Geriatrics Society, 32,* 253–258.

Nagi, S. Z. (1965). Some conceptual issues in disability and rehabilitation. In M. B. Sussman (Ed.), *Sociology and Rehabilitation.* Washington, DC: American Sociological Association.

Ouslander, J. G., & Schnelle, J. F. (1995). Incontinence in the nursing home. *Annals of Internal Medicine, 122(6),* 438–449.

Poon, L. W. (1985). Differences in human memory with aging: Nature, causes and clinical implications. In J. E. Birren, & K. W. Schaie (Eds.), *Handbook of the Psychology of Aging* (2nd ed.). New York: Van Nostrand Reinhold, pp. 427–462.

Ray, W. A., Taylor, J. A., Meador, K. G., Tappa, P. B., Brown, A. K., Davis, C., Gideon, P., & Griffin, M. R. (1997). A randomized trial of a consultation service to reduce falls in nursing homes. *Journal of the American Medical Association, 278(7),* 557–562.

Rentz, D. M. (1991). The assessment of rehabilitation potential: Cognitive factors. In R. J. Hartke (Ed.), *Psychological aspects of geriatric rehabilitation.* Gaithersburg, MD: Aspen.

Rowe, J. W., & Kahn, R. L. (1998). *Successful aging.* New York: Pantheon Books.

Rubenstein, L. Z., Josephson, K. R., Wieland, D., English, P. A., Sayre, J. A., & Kane, R. L. (1984). Effectiveness of a geriatric evaluation unit. *New England Journal of Medicince, 311,* 1664–1670.

Rusk, H. A. (1977). *A world to care for: The autobiography of Howard A. Rusk, M.D.* New York: A Reader's Digest Press Book, Random House.

Schuman, J. E., Beattie, E. J., Steed D. A., Merry G. M., & Kraus, A. S. (1981). Geriatric patients with and without intellectual dysfunction: Effectiveness of a standard rehabilitation program. *Archives of Physical Medicine and Rehabilitation, 62*, 612–618.

Strasser, D. C. (1992). Geriatric rehabilitation: Perspectives from the United Kingdom. *Archives of Physical Medicine and Rehabilitation, 73*, 582–586.

Strasser, D. C. Falconer, J. A., & Martino-Saltzmann, D. (1992). The relationship of patient's age to the perceptions of the the rehabilitation environment. *Journal of the American Geriatrics Society, 40*, 445–448.

Tinetti, M. E., Baker, D. I., McAvay, G., Claus E. B., Garrett, P., Gottschalk, M., Koch, M. L., Trainor, K., & Horwitz, R. I. (1994). A multifactorial intervention to reduce the risk of falling among elderly people living in the community. *New England Journal of Medicine, 331*, 821–827.

U.S. Bureau of the Census, International Population Reports, P25, 92-3. (1992). *An Aging World II.* Washington, DC: U.S. Govemment Printing Office.

Wolf, S. L., Barnhart, H. X., Kutner, N. G., McNeely, E., Coogler, C., Xu, T., & the Atlanta FICSIT Group. (1996). Reducing frailty and falls in older persons: An investigation of Tai Chi and computerized balance training. *Journal of the American Geriatrics Society, 44(5)*, 489–497.

World Health Organization (1999). *ICIDH-2 Beta 2 Draft Introduction.* Assessment, Classification and Epidemiology Group. Geneva, Switzerland: World Health Organization.

Zuckerman, J. D. (1996). Hip fracture. *Current Concepts, New England Journal of Medicine, 334(23)*, 1519–1525.

Psychosocial Considerations in a Rehabilitation Model for Aging and Vision Services

Bryan J. Kemp

Vision loss is a major cause of disability in late life that has profound psychosocial consequences for the older person as well as for his or her family. Vision loss ranks as the third leading reason for an individual to need help with basic activities of daily living (ADLs) in late life and the fourth leading cause of activity limitation (Pope & Tarlov, 1991). When a person first experiences vision loss, community-living skills such as mobility, shopping, managing money, doing chores, and use of household appliances (also known as instrumental activities of daily living, or IADLs) are compromised. As vision worsens, basic living skills such as cooking, dressing, and toileting are often affected. The loss of IADL and ADL skills is a measure of the degree of disability experienced and a good predictor of the person's needs for assistance and even his or her choice of living environment.

The onset of vision loss is also a major cause of *handicap*, defined here as a loss of social roles and social acceptance. The degree of handicap is directly proportional to the difficulties society imposes interpersonally and environmentally. Despite progress in creating a more inclusive environment, visually impaired persons are still excluded from easy access to public streets, buildings, and transportation and still feel a measure of nonacceptance by others.

Rehabilitation is an approach to care and a set of practice principles to help reduce disability—defined as an imbalance between the demands of a task and a person's abilities—and handicap. Rehabilitation's approach values independence, self-sufficiency, and autonomy for people with disability, including those with low vision, whose vision loss cannot be corrected with eyeglasses and is severe enough to interfere with everyday activities. How to accomplish that in the face of a severe disabling condition, a challenging environment, and an as yet noninclusive society is the task of rehabilitation. This chapter briefly describes the basic principles of rehabilitation and describes how older persons differ from younger persons in regard to rehabilitation. Those sections are followed by a discussion of three important psychosocial issues in rehabilitation: the role of depression and other mental health problems that frequently accompany vision loss, maintaining quality of life after vision loss, and the role of the family in the long-term success of the older visually impaired person.

PRINCIPLES OF REHABILITATION

The orientation of rehabilitation toward care and assistance rests on three important principles. The first is that *the person's daily functioning is the primary objective of care.* Functioning usually includes four components: work or avocational activity; instrumental activities of daily living; basic activities of daily living; and the four functional substrates of activity: endurance, strength, coordination, and range of motion. Regardless of the person's underlying impairment (such as low vision, spinal cord injury, or mental illness), function and improving function are the ultimate objectives. In fact, rehabilitation success is measured in terms of functional outcomes achieved and its cost is even reimbursed by government and private insurances on this basis (see Fuhrer, 1997).

The second important principle of rehabilitation is that *function is the product of biological, psychological, and social forces working together.* (See Figure 1.) This is sometimes referred to as the *biopsychosocial*

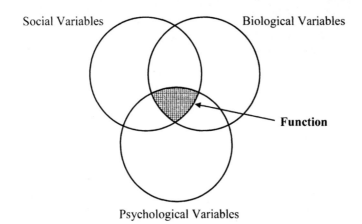

Social Variables

Biological Variables

Function

Psychological Variables

Figure 1
Biological, Psychological, and Social Factors That Influence Function

perspective. An important aspect of this principle is that a variety of physical, psychological, and social factors usually contribute to the person's loss of functioning. Typical physical causes of dysfunction are the primary impairment (such as the illness causing the low vision), but secondary conditions such as diabetes or heart disease, physical deconditioning, or drugs that may cause significant side effects also contribute to dysfunction. Typical psychological causes of dysfunction include depression or other mental health problems, changes in self-esteem or self-confidence, and difficulties with motivation or with learning new ways of doing things. Common social factors affecting function include difficulties in family relationships, lack of economic resources, or environmental obstacles such as poor housing.

The third important principle of rehabilitation is that *improvements in rehabilitation come about in two ways: either by removing the barriers that prevent better function (such as an inappropriate drug), or by providing therapies to improve function (such as physical therapy, occupational therapy, speech therapy, and recreation therapy) or, as usually is the case, by doing both.* When rehabilitation fails, it is usually because the obstacles to rehabilitation cannot be adequately overcome, either because they are undetected (and therefore untreated) or because they are so severe that they can't be overcome. Similarly, when rehabilitation is successful, it is because any existing barrier can be overcome and because

Table 1
Steps in the Practice of Rehabilitation

Practices That Remove Obstacles	*Practices That Improve Function*
1. Stabilizing primary impairment	
2. Preventing or treating secondary conditions	
3. Treating psychological factors	
	4. Providing functional therapies
	5. Modifying the task or environment
6. Treating family problems	
	7. Educating family
	8. Long-term care
	9. Social integration

therapy does improve functioning. Table 1 summarizes the steps comprising rehabilitation practice, and the discussion that follows elaborates on these steps.

Stabilizing the Underlying Impairment

Stabilizing the underlying impairment responsible for the low vision is the essential first step in removing obstacles to better functioning. If the underlying illness is diabetes, which is causing diabetic retinopathy, the diabetes must be brought under control. If the cause is glaucoma, then the intraocular pressure must be treated. Managing the underlying condition is important to prevent a worsening, progressive illness that will then make rehabilitation more difficult and lower the ultimate level of functioning.

Preventing or Treating Secondary Conditions

Secondary conditions, including medical, physical, or psychological problems, are common following a major medical impairment.

Diabetes, which causes low vision, for example, also increases the risk of heart disease, deconditioning due to fatigue or illness, and discouragement stemming from the change of lifestyle. Falls are a common secondary condition to low vision (Tobis et al., 1990). In one year, more than 25 percent of people with low vision fall, often sustaining an injury. Secondary conditions, which are usually preventable, greatly impede rehabilitation and are often the culprit in failed rehabilitation. They must either be prevented or treated aggressively.

Treating Psychological Disorders

Psychological distress, in the form of depression and other disorders, is more common among persons with disability than in the nondisabled population. Depression is a major obstacle to improved function and one that must be carefully assessed and treated. Vision loss does not cause increased psychological problems directly. Rather, these problems are the result of difficulties in coping with the loss because of inadequate social support, prior poor functioning, and the impact of the vision loss on valued activities. The most common psychological disorder following vision loss is depression, which is discussed later in this chapter. Depression itself is disabling, even at moderate levels in nondisabled persons (Judd, Paulus, Wells, & Rapaport, 1996) and is very disabling when it occurs in conjunction with low vision.

Providing Therapy to Improve Function

The provision of various function-improving therapies distinguishes rehabilitation from primary medical care. Individuals with low vision require the assistance of orientation and mobility instructors, rehabilitation teachers, occupational therapists, recreation therapists, physical therapists, and social workers in order to improve physical functioning, basic living skills, community living skills, work skills, and social skills.

Modifying the Task or the Environment

In addition to increasing the person's functional ability, assistance can take the form of altering the task to be performed. Recall that a disability is defined as an imbalance between the demands of a task and a person's abilities to perform on it. Rehabilitation therapies can help restore the imbalance by simplifying the task. Examples from low vision rehabilitation would be the provision of a Kurzweill Reader to make reading easier, the installation of speakers at street corners to orient the person with low vision about his or her location, or the installation of grab bars in the shower to help prevent falls.

Educating Families and Treating Family Problems

Families are a critical element of all rehabilitation practice. (See Chapter 7 for a detailed discussion.) They provide the majority of practical assistance to individuals with a disability as well as the necessary encouragement, support, companionship, and affection. Rehabilitation efforts therefore need to include the family as part of the treatment team. Families may also be a source of difficulty to the person disabled by low vision. Families can lack information about low vision or rehabilitation, feel burdened by the need to provide care, experience conflict, or behave dysfunctionally. Moore (1984) studied 108 adults who were blind and visually impaired and in vocational rehabilitation. Each person was asked to rate his or her family's attitude, and the results were assessed using a semantic differential scale. Far more individuals who rated their families most cohesive and supportive obtained employment compared to persons with less supportive families. Oppegard et al. (1984) found that among older persons with vision loss, social support served as a buffer against depression and anxiety.

Assessment, education, and counseling for families are always needed in rehabilitation. Typically, social workers and rehabilitation therapists provide the majority of these services, with social workers dealing with the more problematic aspects of families and family dynamics and rehabilitation therapists providing education. Clearly, psychosocial issues of the person with vision loss and his or her family are critical to long-term success in rehabilitation.

Providing Long-Term Care

Long-term success in living with a disability also depends on two final requirements: the provision of long-term care services and social integration of the older person with vision loss. Long-term care services are those designed to help the person continue living independently in the community and include primary health care, transportation services, personal assistance services (when needed), financial assistance, and housing. Of these, personal assistance services are the most critical. Assistance in the home can keep individuals independent and out of institutions providing higher levels of care such as residential care facilities or nursing homes.

Fostering Social Acceptance and Integration

Social acceptance of the person who is visually impaired is ultimately a social issue that is the responsibility of society as a whole, not just of rehabilitation professionals. Social acceptance for a person with a disability is part of acceptance of diversity in general. Thus, acceptance is increased when diversity is valued (not just tolerated), when the media include persons with disabilities in general presentations (such as movies and commercials), and when communities include persons with disabilities in all their activities.

HOW OLDER PERSONS ARE DIFFERENT IN REHABILITATION

Older persons are distinctively different from younger persons in regard to their experience of rehabilitation practice. Each of the basic principles and processes described is altered to some degree when the patient is older, especially over the age of 70. At the same time, evidence indicates that when general rehabilitation principles and practices are correctly followed, there are no differences in general rehabilitation outcomes in terms of age (Kemp, Brummel-Smith, & Ramsdell, 1990).

Rehabilitation for older persons still follows a biopsychosocial approach. However, a large difference exists in the degree of interplay among biological, psychological, and social factors. This interplay is greater in late life than it is in younger years. For example, a urinary tract infection in a 75-year-old woman can have profound effects not only symptomatically, but also on function and cognitive status. This interplay is much less likely to occur in younger persons. Likewise, small changes in health or psychological state may lead to a significant change in function for the older person. An older person whose depression is adequately treated, even if it were "only" moderate depression, may show a major improvement in daily functioning. The elimination of an offending drug, or even a reduction in dosage, may lead to a major change in functioning. This increased interdependency among biological, psychological, social, and functional variables is a hallmark of the aging process.

Older persons are also different from younger persons on each of the specific steps in rehabilitation. Older persons typically have multiple chronic illnesses that contribute to their disability, not just one as is typical of younger persons. Older persons have twice the rate of secondary conditions compared to younger persons (Kane, Ouslander, & Abrass, 1989). Thus, for example, the older visually impaired person is more likely to develop deconditioning because of both decreased mobility caused by the low vision and decreased cardiovascular fitness due to age.

Functionally, older persons may need more time to learn the skills necessary to be mobile with low vision or to learn independent living skills because of age-related learning changes. However, changes in teaching techniques can help ameliorate these learning differences, for example, providing more frequent but less lengthy training sessions, more feedback, and increased reassurance (Birren & Schaie, 1985). Older persons who have disability-causing impairments appear to have more psychological problems compared to younger persons (Reinhardt, 1996). This is the result not of age *per se* but rather of the fact that the vision loss is often one of a number of losses the person has experienced over a relatively short period of time.

In addition, although the family of the older person is, if anything, more critical in terms of long-term success, at the same time, the relationship with the family may become even more fraught with difficulties. Families who provide support to older persons are often adult children or spouses. The adult children typically do not reside with the older person, making it difficult to provide day-to-day assistance. Spouses may have their own health problems. The families of older persons usually do not understand what the older person is now capable of and invariably need education so that they do not overly handicap the older person. Although most families resolve these issues, many families are in conflict among themselves as to how to proceed (especially if the older person lives alone), many feel burdened, and most lack information about community resources that could be of assistance to them. Therefore, it becomes impossible to practice good geriatric rehabilitation without a strong program of assessment and assistance for the family.

Finally, long-term care for the older person requires a combination of housing assistance, personal care help, supportive services, and often assistive technology. However, older persons are often uncomfortable managing in-home help, and as up to one-third of older persons live in poverty, housing and basic necessities are often difficult to obtain. Thus, every aspect of rehabilitation practice needs to be adjusted to accommodate older persons.

PSYCHOSOCIAL FACTORS IN VISION REHABILITATION

Psychosocial factors come into play in three primary ways in vision rehabilitation with older persons:

1. *Psychological disorders concomitant to vision loss represent substantial barriers to rehabilitation.* When all psychological disorders are considered, they represent perhaps a third of the obstacles to

successful vision rehabilitation, the others being medical and socioeconomic.

2. *Enhancing the quality of life or life satisfacation essentially determined by psychological phenomena, represents one of the most important outcomes of rehabilitation.* In fact, it can be argued that maintaining health, improving function, and having a high quality of life *are* the three most important outcomes.

3. *Family issues represent the most important psychosocial factors, aside from those affecting the older person himself or herself.* Families can "make or break" rehabilitation efforts. The family's assistance, comfort, and support are key factors in success, whereas any disharmony, incapacity, or dysfunction can undermine all rehabilitation efforts.

These three factors are discussed in more detail in the following sections.

Psychological Disorders

Although a variety of psychological problems may accompany vision loss, including anxiety, substance abuse, and psychosis, by far the most common disorder is depression. The common element in depressive disorders is a change in mood. In older persons, this mood change can be experienced as sadness but can just as likely be expressed as irritability or apathy, often making depression difficult to detect. Besides mood, depression also includes symptoms that reflect changes in thinking (such as a change in outlook or thinking or memory ability), a change in behavior (difficulty relating to others, not looking after oneself, few pleasurable activities, and so on), and changes in physiology (poor sleep, fatigue, lack of ambition, digestive problems, etc.). Depressive disorders encompass a wide range in terms of the severity of symptoms, from relatively mild to major.

Studies of older persons in general indicate that even moderate depression causes loss of functioning and poor interpersonal relationships (Judd et al., 1996). Depressive disorders that are either moderate or severe in terms of diagnostic criteria have a major effect on the older person's health and functioning. Although data are lacking in vision rehabilitation, evidence from studies of older persons with stroke (Morris, Robinson, Andrzejewski, Samuels, & Price, 1993), polio, and spinal cord injury (Kemp, Adams, & Campbell, 1997) indicate increased mortality and about a 33 percent decrease in functioning within 10 years among those who are depressed.

Depressive disorders have been found to be quite common among persons with low vision. Rates are even higher among older persons with low vision and highest among older persons with low vision and other risk factors, including, living alone, other health problems, and poverty (Horowitz, 1995). Fitzgerald, Ebert, and Chambers (1987) found that shortly following the onset of vision loss, 85 percent of people developed significant depressive symptoms. Four years later, 50 percent still had significant symptoms. Others, including Evans (1983) and Horowitz (1995), have reported results similar to these.

The causes of depression are complex. However, it is clear, not only in vision rehabilitation but also in rehabilitation in general, that contrary to what might be expected, depression does not relate to the severity of the impairment or to the duration of the impairment. (See Grieg, West, & Overbury, 1986, and Horowitz, 1995, for evidence on vision; Fuhrer, Rintala, Hart, Clearman, & Young, 1993, for evidence on spinal cord injury; and Kemp, Adams, and Campbell, 1997, for evidence on polio.) Thus, blindness or low vision does not "cause" depression, and depression is not "normal" following low vision.

What, then, causes persons who are visually impaired to be more likely to develop depression? An answer to this can be proposed based on research on stress and coping in general (Folkman, Lazarus, Pintey, & Novacek, 1987; Haley, Levine, Brown, & Santolvicci, 1987; Lazarus & Folkman, 1984; and others). A generalized model of coping has been used to help explain the development of depression in older persons coping with Alzheimer's disease in a spouse (Haley, Levine, Brown, & Santolvicci, 1987) and other conditions.

This model explains depression psychologically as a breakdown in coping. The coping process can be thought of as beginning with the onset of negative life events and involving the way that the person

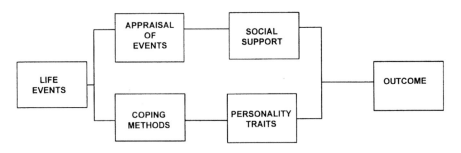

Figure 2
Model of Stress and Coping

appraises (interprets) those events, his or her prior personality, the actual coping methods used, and the degree of social support received. (See Figure 2.)

Numerous studies demonstrate that depression is correlated with various aspects of the coping process (Cairns & Baker, 1993; Fuhrer, 1995; Kemp, 1990; Krause, 1998; Morris et al., 1993; Reinhardt, 1996). The likelihood that a person will become depressed is greatly increased if the following conditions are present:

- The negative events in life are multiple or lead to loss of valued roles or self-esteem.
- The person interprets the events in an extreme manner (such as "catastrophic," "disastrous," or as injurious to self-esteem).
- The person has prior personality traits that are problematic.
- The person receives little or negative social support.
- The person uses ineffective coping methods.

When depression reaches major proportions (e.g., a major depressive episode), then biochemical and psychological processes begin to break down. Biochemical changes involving the neurotransmitters norepinephrine, serotonin, and dopamine alter brain functioning. These neurochemical changes make it very difficult for the depressed person to pull himself or herself out of the depression without the help of medication. The development of significant process symptoms of depression distinguishes major depression from moderate and minor depression. Taken together, difficulties in coping psychologically and the neurochemical changes help account for most depressive disorders.

Horowitz (1995) reported that severity of vision loss was related not to depression but rather to several aspects of the coping process. Lower perceived social support was associated with higher depression. Reinhardt (1996) found that friendship support operated independently from and in addition to family support to serve as a buffer against depression in persons with low vision. Other aspects of the coping model need further investigation in vision rehabilitation research.

Fortunately, the treatment of depression for older persons is both effective and reasonably fast. Most persons begin to improve in a few weeks and are maximally helped within about six to eight months. Moderate depression responds to psychotherapy and a variety of counseling and environmental interventions. Major depressive episodes, because they involve changes in brain neurochemistry and neuropsychological processes, just about always are benefited best by a combination of psychotherapy and antidepressant medicine.

The biggest problem in treatment of depression is still the proper identification, assessment, and differential diagnosis of older persons who are depressed. Although the best assessment method is a clinical interview, screening instruments such as the Geriatric Depression Scale (Yesavage et al., 1983) can be helpful. Another instrument, the Older Adult Health and Mood Questionnaire (Kemp & Adams, 1995) is reproduced in Figure 3. The odd-numbered questions all relate to dysphonic mood, whereas all the even-numbered items relate to cognitive, behavioral, or physiological symptoms of depression that are usually common in older persons. Scores are based on the number of questions answered "true." Scores from 0 to 5 usually indicate no or only low levels of depression, whereas scores from 6 to 10 indicate moderate depressive disorder, and scores of 11 or above indicate a high likelihood of major depression.

Following discovery that someone possibly has a depressive disorder, care should be taken to rule out other causes of these symptoms, including medical, neurological, and pharmacological causes. A

1. My daily life is not interesting.	T or F
2. It is hard for me to get started on my daily chores and activities.	T or F
3. I have been more unhappy than usual for at least a month.	T or F
4. I have been sleeping poorly for at least the last month.	T or F
5. I gain little pleasure from anything.	T or F
6. I feel listless, tired, or fatigued a lot of the time.	T or F
7. I have felt sad or blue much of the time during the last month.	T or F
8. My memory or thinking is not as good as usual.	T or F
9. I have been more easily irritated or frustrated lately.	T or F
10. I feel worse in the morning than in the afternoon.	T or F
11. I have cried or felt like crying more than twice during the last month.	T or F
12. I am definitely slowed down compared to my usual way of feeling.	T or F
13. The things that used to make me happy don't do so anymore.	T or F
14. My appetite or digestion of food is worse than usual.	T or F
15. I frequently feel like I don't care about anything anymore.	T or F
16. Life is really not worth living most of the time.	T or F
17. My outlook is more gloomy than usual.	T or F
18. I have stopped several of my usual activities.	T or F
19. I cry or feel saddened more easily than a few months ago.	T or F
20. I feel pretty hopeless about improving.	T or F
21. I seem to have lost the ability to have any fun.	T or F
22. I have regrets about the past that I think about often.	T or F

Figure 3
Older Adult Health and Mood Questionnaire

Source: Kemp, B. J., & Adams, B. M. (1995). The older adult health and mood questionnaire: A measure of geriatric depressive disorder. *Journal of Geriatric Psychiatry and Neurology, 8,* 162–167.

variety of medical conditions can mimic depression, including hypothyroidism, heart disease, anemia, infections, dementia, cancer, and diabetes. Drugs that are frequently prescribed for older persons, including antihypertensive, anxiolitic, antiinflammatory, and antiarrhythmic agents, can cause depression-like symptoms.

Psychotherapy of the cognitive–behavioral kind (Gallagher-Thompson, Lovett, Rose, & Futterman, 1993) is effective for older adults. This kind of therapy focuses on the irrational cognitive or behavioral elements that cause and sustain depression. For example, most depressed persons have thoughts such as "Life is over for me," "Things will never get better," or "I'm such a burden," that serve to maintain depressive feelings. They also do not engage in pleasurable activities or flexible problem-solving that would lead to more positive feelings and successful interpersonal relationships. Other problem-solving and supportive methods may also help. Evans, Werkhoven, and Fox (1982) conducted telephone counseling sessions with older visually impaired adults who were moderately depressed. Their results showed that eight one-hour group conference call sessions involving up to three persons was effective in reducing depressive symptoms, increasing activity levels, and promoting higher self-acceptance.

Antidepressant medicines also greatly aid the treatment of depression. Most experts would suggest both antidepressant medicine and psychotherapy for persons with major depression—medicine to help restore basic brain processes and psychotherapy to promote better problem-solving and long-term adjustments. Among the many antidepressants available, a few are used more often with older persons because they have fewer side effects. For example, Paxil and Zoloft have proven effective in treatment of older persons, and Pamelor, Norpramin, and Desyrel are among the safer older medications.

Quality-of-Life Issues

The second way that psychosocial factors enter into rehabilitation is in the form of quality-of-life issues. Quality of life can be measured on a continuum. On the lower end of a quality-of-life scale is distress, depression, and despair with associated poor health and poor daily functioning. On the upper end is life satisfaction, with accompanying good health and good functioning. In the middle is neither distress nor satisfaction but rather feelings of "getting by," boredom, or lack of direction. Measures of depression and measures of life satisfaction can be used to assess the anchor points on quality of life. Depression and life satisfaction scales are therefore moderately negatively correlated with each other. Reinhardt (1996), for example, found that her measures of health, functioning, and support had opposite relationships with depression than they had with life satisfaction. She found that among 241 older persons experiencing vision loss, life satisfaction scores averaged only 9.7 on an 18-point scale, below the average for nondisabled older persons. Higher scores on life satisfaction were associated with a higher quality of friendship, a higher degree of family support, and greater independence.

Findings from numerous studies (Cairns & Baker, 1993; Fuhrer, 1995; Kemp, 1990; Krause, 1998; Morris et al., 1993; Reinhardt, 1996), when taken together, suggest a two-factor model of quality-of-life. The first factor accounts for low quality-of-life, as reflected in distress, despair, and depression. This factor is described as inability to cope with the changes brought about by the vision loss. The variables in the model of coping described earlier are the critical ones in this factor. Improving depression and distress focuses on enhancing coping abilities by developing better methods of coping, adopting a different outlook about the loss, utilizing social support, and eliminating self-defeating behaviors. However, the reduction of distress and depression will not result by itself in a high quality of life, in less distress.

The second factor in this model of quality of life is what moves the person from a state of not being distressed to true life satisfaction. Here the critical factor appears to be maintaining valued activities. Three kinds of activities are valued—those that provide

- ♦ Pleasure (enjoyment, fun)
- ♦ Success (achievement, income)
- ♦ Meaning (social roles, purpose, a reason for living)

Data from groups of people with various impairments show that life satisfaction is unrelated to the severity of impairment (such as degree of paralysis or extent of vision loss), degree of ADL disability, age, or duration of disability, but is related to work, social role performance, and recreation (Fuhrer, 1996; Kemp, Brummel-Smith, & Ramsdell, 1990; Krause, 1998).

Older persons with low vision have both higher levels of depression, as already noted, and lower levels of life satisfaction compared to nondisabled older persons. The reasons for this are, as predicted, not directly attributable to the vision loss. Rather, they reflect the difficulties people have coping with vision loss and the additional difficulties they have achieving a reasonable amount of pleasure, success, and meaning in life to compensate for the loss. Future studies in this area need to include a unique measure of pleasurable, successful, and meaningful experiences to test whether they added to life satisfaction. The area of quality of life needs much more research to help understand the impact of vision loss on older persons.

Family Issues

The third major psychosocial factor in rehabilitation is the role of the family. A disability in later life seems to bring out both the best and the worst in families, not only because it is a source of stress but because it brings forth issues about dependency, aging, and autonomy that are new to most families. Families frequently are not really concerned about the autonomy of an older person until a disability occurs. Then issues relating to the disability or to previously existing family problems surface, often in extreme forms, because of the stress a disability produces on the family unit.

In unpublished studies of families done at Rancho Los Amigos Medical Center involving older persons with a variety of impairments, many involving vision, it was discovered that over 60 percent of families had a problem that was significant enough to affect the older person's rehabilitation and independence. In trying to assess these families and to characterize their dynamics, a four-part rating was used. Families were rated on support for each other, cohesiveness, resourcefulness, and affection. Simple three-point scaling (low, medium, high) was enough to distinguish families clinically. Across all impairments, family functioning was found to relate to patient outcomes to a major extent. Horowitz (1995) reported on studies involving a person with low vision. Higher levels of depression were associated with a lower level of perceived family support. Reinhardt (1996), as noted earlier, found that total family support was positively correlated with life satisfaction ($r = 0.39$) and negatively correlated with depression ($r = -0.31$).

Although family support is indeed important, problems in obtaining support from stressed families and problems in families associated with disability are common. Families may need different types of intervention from professionals, depending on their history and dynamics. Several typical family styles can be observed in geriatrics. The "Healthy Family" is supportive, cohesive, resourceful, and affectionate with each other and with the older person. They mostly need information about the vision loss, about aging, and about what to expect in the future. With information, they do well at helping themselves.

Two styles of familes need more than information. They need support and counseling. These might be called the "Burdened Family" and the "Conflicted Family." The Burdened Family includes one or more members who are excessively stressed. Perhaps one person takes on disproportionate caregiving responsibilities or has multiple responsibilities for others, such as younger children or work. The Conflicted Family is not cohesive and disagrees about what the care should be for the older person, where he or she should live, and how much independence is possible.

Two styles of families need education, support, and deeper counseling. These are the "Old Business Family" and the "She'll Do It Family." In the former type of family, the impairment to the older person represents a crisis that makes family members confront old issues that were never successfully resolved. This may involve prior problems of the older person (e.g., alcoholism), previous conflicts among siblings, or unresolved family conflicts. The family, now under stress, displays low levels of cohesiveness, support for each other, affection, and resourcefulness. Arguments are likely to increase. Such conflict predicts a poor outcome for the older person. In the "She'll Do It Family," one person, typically a daughter or daughter-in-law, is expected to absorb all the duties and care of the older person. This often results in resentment or anger, with the identified caretaker feeling martyred. Breaking the cycle of those two dysfunctional families may take several months.

For the most part, families do try to do the best they can within the dynamics they have previously developed. Education, support groups, counseling, community services, and family therapy can all contribute to helping the family to better help the older person with vision loss.

CONCLUSION

Geriatric vision rehabilitation is becoming increasingly important. By the year 2020, 80 million people in the United States, or about 18 percent of the total population, will be over the age of 65 (Kane, Ouslander, & Abrass, 1989). Vision problems increase substantially with age and represent a major cause of disability. Rehabilitation is a way of preserving and promoting independence for these persons, but it must be tailored to the older person's unique problems and differences. If these differences, such as the higher rate of secondary conditions, are incorporated into rehabilitation practice, then outcomes for older persons can be as good as those for younger persons. Psychological issues also present important challenges with older persons. In particular, identifying and treating mental health problems and helping to provide a reasonable level of life satisfaction are two critical issues. Depression is a common problem in geriatrics that is in general inadequately identified and inadequately treated. It is most often caused by difficulties in coping with losses, often multiple losses. However, it can be treated with great success. Life satisfaction appears to require maintaining valued and meaningful experiences involving social, family, and purposeful activities. These activities can be maintained in spite of vision loss and will greatly improve the quality of life of older persons.

REFERENCES

Birren, J., & Schaie, W. (1985). *The handbook of the psychology of aging.* New York: Van Nostrand Reinhold.

Cairns, D., & Baker, J. (1993). Adjustment to spinal cord injury: A review of coping styles contributing to the process. *Journal of Rehabilitation, 59,* 30–33.

Evans, R. L. (1983). Loneliness, depression and social activity after determination of legal blindness. *Psychological Reports, 52,* 603–608.

Evans, R. L., Werkhoven, W., & Fox, H. R. (1982). Treatment of social isolation and loneliness in a sample of visually impaired elderly persons. *Psychology Reports, 51,* 103–108.

Fitzgerald, R. G., Ebert, J. N., & Chambers, M. (1987). Reactions to blindness: A four-year follow-up study. *Perceptual and Motor Skills, 64,* 363–378.

Folkman, S., Lazarus, R. S., Pintey, S., & Novacek, J. (1987). Age deficiencies in stress and coping processes. *Psychology and Aging, 2,* 171–184.

Fuhrer, M. (1996). The subjective well-being of people with spinal cord injury: Relationships to impairment, disability and handicap. *Topics In Spinal Cord Injury Rehabilitation, 1,* 56–71.

Fuhrer, M. J. (Ed.) (1997). *Assessing medical rehabilitation practices: The promise of outcomes research.* Baltimore: Brookes.

Fuhrer, M., Rintala, D. H., Hart, K., Clearman, R., & Young, M. E. (1992). Relationship of life satisfaction to impairment, disability and handicap among persons with spinal cord injury living in the community. *Archives of Physical Medicine and Rehabilitation, 73,* 552–557.

Gallagher-Thompson, D., Lovett, S., Rose, J., & Futterman, A. (1993). The impact of psychoeducational interventions on distressed family caregivers. *The Gerontologist, 31,* 151–159.

Greig, D. E., West, M. L., & Overbury, O. (1986). Successful use of low vision aids: Visual and psychological factors. *Journal of Visual Impairment & Blindness, 80*(10), 985–988.

Haley, W. E., Levine, E. G., Brown, J. W., & Santolvicci, A. (1987). Stress appraisal, coping and social support as predictors of adaptational outcome among dementia caregivers. *Psychology and Aging, 2,* 323–330.

Horowitz, A. (1995). Aging, vision loss and depression: A review of the research. *Aging and Vision News, 7*(1), 1, 6–7.

Judd, L. L., Paulus, M. B., Wells, K. B., & Rapaport, M. H. (1996). Socioeconomic burden of subsyndromal depression symptoms and major depression in a sample of the general population. *American Journal of Psychiatry, 153,* 1411–1417.

Kane, R. C., Ouslander, J. G., and Abrass, I. B. 1989. *Essentials of Clinical Geriatrics,* 2nd ed. New York: McGraw-Hill.

Kemp, B., & Adams, B. (1990). The older adult health and mood questionnaire: A measure of geriatric depression disorder. *Geriatric Psychiatry and Neurology, 8,* 162–167.

Kemp, B., Adams, B. & Campbell, M. (1997). Depression and life satisfaction in aging polio survivors versus age matched controls. *Archives of Physical Medicine and Rehabilitation, 78,* 187–192.

Kemp, B., Brummel-Smith, K., & Ramsdell, J. (Eds.) (1990). *Geriatric rehabilitation.* Boston: Little, Brown.

Krause, J. (1998). Longitudinal changes in adjustment after spinal cord injury: A 15-year study. *Archives of Physical Medicine and Rehabilitation, 73,* 564–568.

Lazarus, R. S., & Folkman, S. (1984). Coping and adaptation. In W. D. Gentry, (Ed.) *The handbook of behavioral mechanics.* New York: Guilford.

Moore, J. E. (1984). Impact of family attitudes toward blindness/visual impairment on the rehabilitation process. *Journal of Visual Impairment & Blindness, 78,* 100–106.

Morris, P. L. P., Robinson, R. G., Andrzejewski, M. S., Samuels, J., & Price T. R. (1993). Association of depression with 10-year post-stroke mortality. *American Journal of Psychiatry, 150,* 124–129.

Oppegard, K., Hansson, R. O., Morgan, T., Indart, M., Crutcher, M., & Hampton, P. (1984). Sensory loss, family support, and adjustment among the elderly. *Journal of Social Psychology, 123,* 291–292.

Pope, A. & Tarlov, A. (Eds.) (1991). *Disability in America: Toward a national agenda for prevention.* Washington, DC: National Academy Press.

Reinhardt, J. P. (1996). The importance of friendship and family support in adaptation to chronic vision impairment. *Journal of Gerontology: Psychological Sciences, 51B* (5), 268–278.

Tobis, J. S., Block, M., Steinhaus-Donham, C., Reinsch, S., Tamura, K., & Weil, D. (1990). Falling among the sensorially impaired elderly. *Archives of Physical Medicine and Rehabilitation, 71,* 144–147.

Yesavage, Y. A., Brink, T. L., Rose, T. L., Win, O., Hvong, V., Adex, M. B., & Leirer, V. D. (1983). Development and validation of a geriatric depression screening scale. *Journal of Psychiatric Research, 17,* 37–49.

CHAPTER 7

Aging,
Vision Rehabilitation,
and the Family

Barbara Silverstone

This discussion focuses on the families of older persons with impaired vision. It examines the impact of the older person's vision loss on family members and the role the family plays in the adaptation of the older person to vision impairment and in the rehabilitation process itself. A model of vision rehabilitation is then proposed that embraces the family's needs as well as those of the older person. However, first a review of the status of the family in traditional vision rehabilitation efforts is in order, for the model of vision rehabilitation to be proposed is not universally appreciated or practiced.

It was not long ago that the subjects of aging, families, and rehabilitation were seen as distinct if not unrelated entities. Aging itself is a relatively new subject for study. It was not until the latter half of the twentieth century, with the dramatic growth in the aging population, that a body of knowledge about aging and aging populations was accumulated. The family life of older people, however, received short shrift from gerontologists in early research. Families were viewed as largely irrelevant to the aging process, and older people for the most part were assumed to be without families or isolated from them.

It was only in the past 30 years that researchers documented through extensive surveys that most older people were deeply embedded in rich and reciprocal intergenerational family relationships and that families of older people were important if not critical sources of support in their lives (e.g., Shanas, 1979). Interest on the part of the gerontological community in family caregiving mushroomed when it was recognized that the bulk of long-term care to frail older people was provided by the informal network. The stresses experienced by families caring for older persons with dementia has been of particular concern (Rabins, Mace, & Lucas, 1982).

Beginning in the early 1980s, dementia captured center stage as a disabling condition occurring in late life, and, until recently, gerontologists gave little attention to other disabilities, the benefits of rehabilitation in relation to these disabilities, or the role played by families (Brody, 1985). Thanks to pioneers such as Bryan Kemp (1986), T. Franklin Williams (1984), and Stanley Brody (1986), the field of aging is now moving beyond an emphasis on interventions to protect and support disabled older people toward interventions that enhance independent functioning. More attention also is being given to the discrete components of disability in later life such as vision impairment, which, alone or in combination with other age-related conditions, can result in functional dependency. In addition, studies of the adaptations to vision impairment made by older people are being reported in the literature (Horowitz, Silverstone, & Reinhardt, 1991; Silverstone, 1993). Also encouraging is the increasing interest on the part of the general rehabilitation research community in age-related disabilities and the role played by families (Kaufman, Albright, & Wagner, 1987).

The past reluctance of the gerontological community to foster geriatric rehabilitation and view the family in a context broader than intensive hands-on caregiving was reinforced by a reluctant vision rehabilitation community. Here, programs favor younger persons and those who are career bound, a bias that is understandable given the fact that government reimbursement for the most part targets vocational rehabilitation. A lack of comprehensive coverage for the full range of vision rehabilitation services to people of all ages has been a major roadblock to the development of services to older people. Some strides are being made with the support of philanthropic funding, and, to a limited degree, under Title VII, Chapter 2, of the Rehabilitation Act, which provides federal funding for independent living services to older individauls who are blind or visually impaired (Rogers & Long, 1991). Still, vision rehabilitation services for older people have yet to be fully embraced by the field (Lidoff, 1997). In those agencies providing services to older people, the focus usually is exclusively on the individual—a practice in keeping with the traditional model of vocational rehabilitation and its standard protocol, the Individualized Written Rehabilitation Plan mandated by federal funding legislation and outlining objectives to be met and services to be provided (Crews, 1991). This focus reflects the independent living movement of the 1960s that championed the needs of younger adults to live independently of caregivers, including the family.

Thus, we are dealing with a subject—involving families in the rehabilitation of visually impaired older persons—that is obscure. Older people who have incurred age-related vision loss, and especially their families, have, until recently, fallen through the cracks as subjects for study and recipients of service, and the role of families in the lives of visually impaired older people as well as their rehabilitation is not well known. However, extrapolating from extensive gerontological research on the family, generic rehabilitation studies, and several recent studies of the informal networks of older visually impaired persons, we can construct a viable model of family-oriented vision rehabilitation for older people that lends itself to clinical and empirical validation. This chapter summarizes these findings and presents such a model.

THE IMPORTANCE OF SOCIAL SUPPORTS

As noted, the importance of family, friends, and neighbors in the lives of older people has been well established. Most older people are well integrated into social networks and report substantial contact with children, grandchildren, and friends. More than 75 percent of older men (65 years and over) and 40 percent of older women live with a spouse. Six percent of men and 17 percent of women live with their children or another relative. Most elders who live alone are in near proximity to at least one child or other relative with whom they have regular contact (Administration on Aging, 1996).

The relationships of older people with their extended family have been found to be generally strong on several dimensions, including affectional ties and the exchange of goods and services (Bengtson & Kuypers, 1971). When illness and disability strike, the family is the first and at times the only line of support for older people. A hierarchical progression of support for older people has been described, starting with the spouse, if present, filling the role of primary caregiver; the adult children filling this role if the spouse is not present or functional; and lastly, friends and neighbors (Cantor & Little, 1985). Family caregiving is such a significant support in the lives of chronically impaired older people that the weakening or absence of this support has been found to be an important predictor of nursing home placement (Horowitz, 1985).

Family caregiving of disabled or ill older people is multifaceted, ranging from occasional intermittent assistance with a variety of daily tasks, including household needs or chauffeuring, to 24-hour hands-on caregiving. Studies have also identified emotional support and assistance in negotiating formal systems as important family tasks (Cicerelli, 1983). Friends often fill the role of confidant and emotional supporter and sometimes are preferred to relatives (Reinhardt, 1996).

It is not surprising, therefore, that a close relationship exists between mental and physical well-being among older people and the extent and quality of their social supports (Antonucci, 1990). As older people face the developmental tasks of aging, which include maintaining quality and continuity of life in the face of increased disability and illness, the family can be an important mitigating force, and there is no reason to assume that this is less true for older people with impaired vision.

It is also not surprising that the lives of family members have been found to be affected by the caregiving role they play in relation to a chronically impaired aging relative. Much of the family research conducted to date has focused on the burden and impact of stress experienced from providing care to a relative with a chronic mental impairment, usually Alzheimer's disease (Barer & Johnson, 1990). Findings suggest that the caregiver most likely to exhibit signs of physical and mental stress is the female spouse or others involved in intensive daily care. The emotional component of caregiving is reported to be the greatest burden experienced by family members, surpassing difficult hands-on duties (Cantor, 1983). Interestingly, in spite of these burdens, many family members report positive benefits from the caregiving role in the satisfaction they experience in fulfilling filial responsibilities (Reece, Walz, & Hageboeck, 1983).

THE ROLE OF THE FAMILY IN GERIATRIC REHABILITATION

The role of the family in geriatric rehabilitation has gained increased attention (Brody, 1986). The importance of family involvement and attitudes during the rehabilitation process as well as in the retention of rehabilitation gains is emphasized in the literature. It has been demonstrated that family attitudes are an important factor in the decision to pursue rehabilitation in the first place (Kaufman et al., 1987).

The close relationship between the availability and quality of social supports and positive rehabilitation outcomes has been reported in studies of various physical conditions including stroke, hip fracture, diabetes, and impaired hearing and mobility (Evans, Bishop, & Haselkorn, 1991; McNett, 1987; Oakes et al., 1970; Shenkel, Rogers, Perfeito, & Levin, 1986; Thomas & Stevens, 1974; Weinberger, 1980). In these studies, family support was associated with shorter and improved recoveries, compliance, and better coping mechanisms and adjustment overall. In these and other studies and projects, models of family intervention that have been reported to be effective, primarily based on clinical experience, are support groups, education seminars, literature distribution, family counseling, and direct involvement of families in treatment or rehabilitation sessions.

Studies specifically focused on age-related vision loss and the role of family have yielded similar findings. The overall adjustment of older persons with impaired vision has been significantly associated with the perceptions, attitudes, and behaviors of family members (Large, 1982). Vision loss associated with depression was found among older people with low social supports but not in those with high support (Oppegard et al., 1984). The quality of the relationship with a close family member, not merely the availability of family, has been identified as a predictor of the older person's adaptation to vision loss (Horowitz & Reinhardt, 1992). A high level of family support has also been found to be associated with successful utilization of low vision optical devices (Grieg, West, & Overbury, 1986).

In summary, a strong body of evidence has been amassed documenting the important supportive role played by the family in the lives of older people and, it would appear, also in the rehabilitation of disabled older people, including those who are visually impaired. Caution is required, however, in designing a family-oriented vision rehabilitation model based solely on this evidence. Unlike the families caring for persons with Alzheimer's disease, little is known about the behaviors of families of older people with physical disabilities, including vision impairment and how families are affected by having to play a supportive role. One of the few studies investigating the impact of age-related vision loss on families revealed high levels of reported stress on the part of families caused by worry about the older person's safety, emotional state, and inability to manage the activities of daily living (Crews & Frey, 1993). Although this study was revealing in its description of a sample of 47 families involved in the rehabilitation of legally blind adults, some with other disabilities as well, it did not speak to the large population of older persons seeking rehabilitation for whom vision impairment is the only reported disability.

A family-oriented vision rehabilitation program requires an understanding of the differential effects of vision loss—as a unique impairing condition—on a broad array of individual and family situations. A research demonstration project conducted at Lighthouse International (formerly The Lighthouse Inc.) provides further clues to understanding the behaviors of the family members of older persons with impaired vision (Horowitz et al., 1998). Several of the clinical observations made during the time of this demonstration (1995–1997) have illuminated the discussion that follows.

AGE-RELATED VISION LOSS

Age-related vision loss is unique in several respects. It bears similarities as well as dissimilarities to other chronic impairing conditions, and it must be assumed that, to some extent, it is experienced differently by older people than by their families. Comparisons to dementia are first in order because of the abundance of research documenting the negative effects on caregivers of persons with Alzheimer's disease, including compromised physical and mental health on the part of the family caregiver. Like dementia, age-related vision loss is significantly associated with reduced ability to perform the activities of daily living and to negotiate the environment (Branch, Horowitz, & Carr, 1989). As in the case of dementia, progression of age-related vision diseases is usually gradual, and depressive symptomatology is frequently exhibited.

The similarities between age-related vision loss and dementia, however, stop here. Unless affected by dementia as well, older persons with age-related vision loss are not cognitively impaired and do not display the confusion and memory loss that are profoundly upsetting to family members. Although recent studies report that vision impairment can affect cognitive functioning to the extent that visual data are not as available to the older person, these effects in no way approach the personality changes associated with dementia.

It is important to note that neither the older person with impaired vision nor his or her family members is coping with the devastating effects on rational communication and interpersonal relations and the ubiquitous negative impact on functioning that dementia brings. The high levels of stress reported by family caregivers of older people with Alzheimer's disease cannot be assumed to occur always or frequently in situations involving age-related vision loss.

The behavior of family members whose older member has incurred an acute medical crisis also cannot be automatically transposed to the case of vision impairment. Heart attacks, strokes, and hip fractures represent medical emergencies, and life-saving interventions are paramount. Although chronic in nature, diabetes also can be viewed as a life-threatening medical condition if left uncontrolled. With the exception of diabetes, the diseases underlying vision impairment are not life threatening, and their course of development is usually progressive and slow in comparison. In fact, it is often difficult for the older individual to discern the boundary between the normal vision changes associated with aging and the early stages of impairing vision diseases (Silverstone, 1993).

Thus, it follows that vision impairment is not necessarily viewed by family members as a crisis requiring their immediate attention. Early signs are often viewed as part of the normal aging process, and small everyday adaptations made by the older person to the gradual loss of vision can quell family concerns. In the family-oriented vision re-habilitation program at Lighthouse International, it was found that in some cases the older person's concern about his or her increasingly poor vision preceded that of the family. These older people sought out vision rehabilitation services without the involvement of actively concerned relatives. Furthermore, some older people did not want to involve family members regardless of the degree of family concern. They did not want to burden their families or invite interference in their lives (Horowitz et al., 1998).

The point to be underscored is that the demonstrated concern and involvement of most families of older people who have other disabling conditions that have been reported in the literature may not always be evident in the case of age-related vision loss. Families may not recognize or be alerted by the older person to the seriousness of the condition. Conditions of partial sight may not be as disturbing as dementia and hearing impairment, which interfere with communication. The proclivity of most human beings to see the best in most situations and deny the worst can more easily be played out in the case of age-related vision loss. This lack of active involvement on the part of families was seen in many cases in the demonstration program at Lighthouse International (Horowitz et al., 1998). Fewer than 20 percent of families participated in group meetings; 41 percent in training. Given the reluctance of some older consumers to involve their families, it must be assumed that they did not view vision loss as a crisis.

There comes a time, however, when at least some families are significantly affected by the vision impairment of an older relative, and in some situations their concerns may precede or be greater than those of the older person. Denial of impaired vision is not uncommon among some older people who continue performing with difficulty activities that are unsafe, the most dramatic example of which is driving an automobile. The depression not infrequently experienced by older people who have vision loss is disturbing to families (Hersen et al., 1995). As noted, one of the few studies that examined the impact on families of having older visually impaired relatives reported on high levels of stress attributable due to worry about the older person's safety, emotional state, and inability to manage the activities of daily living (Crews & Frey, 1993). In Lighthouse International's family-oriented rehabilitation program, nearly 40 percent reported stressful effects from their elder's vision impairment. Furthermore, families who participated in programs providing family support and counseling reported significant benefits. As would be expected, the most highly stressed relatives were those living with, or in close proximity to, the older persons and providing care for them (Horowitz et al., 1998).

In summary, age-related vision loss, in its early stages and unencumbered by other impairing conditions, is not necessarily a stressful circumstance for family members, with the exception of those situations where the older person is depressed or a safety risk. As the Lighthouse experience has shown, this may be the case even when the older person is receiving rehabilitation. Many older persons with impaired vision can function at high levels and their condition need not be viewed as a life-threatening crisis. Not surprisingly, these individuals pride themselves on their independent functioning, a *raison d'être* for seeking rehabilitation in the first place.

There may also be circumstances in which family members living in proximity or with an older person, such as a spouse, have made adaptations with the older person to the vision impairment over time that are acceptable, if not ideal, and may never seek help. Furthermore, many elderly people who have impaired vision and their families are unaware of the benefits of vision rehabilitation, and if a problem is recognized may seek only medical or surgical attention (Lighthouse National Survey, 1995). Such a step does not necessarily lead the family or individual to rehabilitation that can provide functional improvements. Unlike other conditions such as stroke or hip fracture, for which rehabilitation is viewed as mandatory, many vision care professionals do not refer older patients for vision rehabilitation (Greenblatt, 1988).

It follows that a family-oriented vision rehabilitation model for older people must accommodate a wide variety of family situations ranging from families who, from the start, are actively involved in the rehabilitation process to those not even aware of the seriousness of the problem. A complex array of situations reflecting the heterogeneity of older people and their families in general and the unique circumstances of age-related vision loss lies between these extremes.

A FAMILY-ORIENTED VISION REHABILITATION PROGRAM

A model of vision rehabilitation is required that addresses the heterogeneity of family situations. Before elaborating on the components of such a model, organizational issues must be addressed if any type of family-oriented model is to thrive in a rehabilitation setting.

Organizational Issues

A formidable barrier to a family-oriented vision rehabilitation model is *the individualized treatment plan* that is utilized in most agencies and is promulgated by federal funding sources (Crews, 1991). Because funding is based upon individual contacts with the visually impaired client, there are no financial incentives for a broader family-based approach that might incur additional up-front costs (even though in the long run it is likely to be more cost effective). Although there is no substitute for a highly motivated older client who utilizes rehabilitation to the fullest, there are those for whom the benefits of rehabilitation are compromised by family situations, and provisions for meeting with family members should be accommodated in the treatment plan.

For agencies with sufficient resources, an investment in a family-oriented approach to vision rehabilitation is advisable. If funding will not pay for family services, consideration should be given to involving family members in sessions with the visually impaired elder so as not to incur additional costs. Such an approach is often advisable for clinical reasons, as discussed later. In any case, staff efforts to involve families should be rewarded, and rehabilitation agencies interested in implementing a family-oriented program must commit the necessary resources.

Not to be overlooked in the implementation of a family-oriented program is the need for enriched in-service training in family dynamics and family counseling in addition to content on the psychology of aging. This ongoing in-service training should be provided to all members of the rehabilitation team—not only the social workers or counselors. Clinical situations regarding older people alone or older people and their families are rarely simple ones, and if a program is to be effective, then resources must be allocated to in-service training.

Another barrier to involving families in the rehabilitation process is the commitment of professionals to *client self-determination.* In particular, concerns have grown in the gerontological community about the impact of actions by family members and formal caregivers that might compromise the autonomy of vulnerable older people (Hofland, 1988). Social workers, particularly if they serve as counselors and case managers in rehabilitation settings, are unwilling for ethical reasons to involve families unless the older person agrees to this. Clearly, contact with families should not be made if prohibited by the older person, but this ethical consideration can be applied too rigidly, resulting in a failure to try even to understand the older person's reluctance to involve family members or to explore family issues. Behind the reluctance may be a serious family situation that warrants professional attention. Given the fact that many older people are accompanied by a relative to the vision rehabilitation setting and, as the research shows, are often concerned about the elder's autonomy (Horowitz et al., 1991), a proactive family approach is warranted. As discussed later, a sensitive clinical approach can reconcile the older client's right to self-determination with productive involvement of family members.

Required in any setting is an open discussion on all administrative and staff levels of the organizational issues that can stand in the way of a family-oriented approach to vision rehabilitation. Without this commitment, such a model will be difficult, if not impossible, to implement. With a full organizational commitment to a family-oriented model, however, a flexible range of services and programs can be offered, depending on the needs of the visually impaired older person and his or her family.

The Family Assessment

The general assessment that initiates any rehabilitation program provides an opportunity for "sizing up" the older person with a visual impairment, not only in terms of individual issues but also within the context of his or her social environment. To be considered are cultural and economic factors that bear upon the older person's adaptation to vision loss and the informal supports available to him or her. Family behavior patterns can vary among different ethnic groups. Of particular importance are family attitudes about disability, seeking and receiving assistance, and caregiving. The heterogeneity of family situations has already been underscored. However, these situations fall into three broad categories that can provide a framework for a systematic assessment of the family situation:

1. The older person's concern about his or her vision loss is greater than that of the family, or he or she does not want the family involved.
2. The family of the older person is concerned with the vision loss but does not perceive a crisis.
3. The family is experiencing a crisis in relation to the older person's vision loss and often experiences a great deal of stress.

Usually, information about the physical environment and the consumer's difficulty in accessing it visually is forthcoming. This information is critical for understanding the special challenges facing the consumers and must be pursued, but it also can be expanded to the social arena. Rarely is the presenting problem of vision loss discussed by a consumer without reference to the people he or she interacts with on a daily basis. If these are family members, the type of family situation can easily be identified. If family members are omitted from discussion, inquiries can be made about the omission to ascertain the type of family situation, as in the following situation:

Seventy-five-year-old Mrs. C., who came alone to the interview, told the intake worker that she was no longer able to read and that her eye care doctor, who diagnosed macular degeneration, suggested she seek vision rehabilitation services. After seeking and receiving more information about Mrs. C.'s vision impairment, the worker asked how she was managing at home. Mrs. C. started to cry and said that she was now having difficulty cooking and shopping and had a few friends and neighbors who helped her out. She was eager for training so that she could continue living on her own. The worker asked if she had family members she could turn to. Mrs. C. became even more upset as she then spoke of her son who lived 20 miles away. She said he was a "good son" and called often but was having serious problems with his wife, who was receiving chemotherapy following a mastectomy. Mrs. C. felt it was her role to support him, not vice versa, and thus had not shared with him the extent of her vision problems.

Mrs. C.'s story unfolded quickly with only a few questions from the intake worker. Within a few minutes, it became apparent that this was a troubled family situation that had to be factored into the rehabilitation equation.

Rarely does an older person refuse to speak about their family situation; more likely, those who refrain from mentioning their families are not ready to involve them. This dynamic is particularly true of some older people who seek rehabilitation in order to maintain an independent lifestyle that they fear will be jeopardized by family involvement. In these situations, as borne out in Lighthouse International experience, appropriate timing is important. For example, premature efforts to involve Mrs. C.'s son might have forced the older client to step back from talking about her family. It is far more important to understand the family situation from the older person's perspective than to involve family members before the older person is ready.

If, on the other hand, family members are readily available, such as those who accompany an older person to the intake interview or are present when a home visit is made, the worker has an excellent opportunity to observe family dynamics first-hand and to hear the perspective of family members. Whenever the family is engaged, the worker should assess the need on the part of family members for emotional support—a need that may supersede that for information.

Although meeting with family members and the older person together is productive, it might be advisable also to speak alone with the older person if, in the judgment of the worker, the client's own perspective has not been aired, as in the case of Mr. P.:

Ninety-year-old Mr. P. was accompanied by his daughter, who lived with him in a two-family house, with Mr. P. occupying the lower floor. The daughter spoke anxiously about Mr. P.'s condition and the growing concerns of his family. Clearly, she was more anxious than the father, so the worker decided to meet with him alone. Alone, Mr. P. spoke affectionately about his daughter and family but was feeling increasingly smothered by them since his wife's death two years ago. His failing vision only made matters worse. He was hoping to do more things on his own but didn't want to hurt his daughter's feelings.

If the assessment interview can be seen as a time for the client to tell his or her story, the family situation will unfold along with other important facts about the client. By inserting questions here and there with the flow of the story and making sure that the client is telling his story, as in the case of Mr. P., the family situation can be "sized up," at least to the extent that the family situation is assessed and an appropriate intervention plan initiated.

The Plan

A variety of programs and services have been successfully offered to families of disabled older adults, either for the purpose of involving them in the rehabilitation process or helping to improve problematic family situations. For situations in which family involvement appears appropriate (i.e., the older person is ready and agrees to involvement), these interventions include the distribution of educational materials, family attendance at open houses, educational forums, support groups for families with or without the older person, or individual and family group meetings. The type of family situation will determine the appropriate intervention and its timing.

Information

It should be assumed from survey findings that all families need more information about visual impairment, regardless of their degree of concern or involvement (Lighthouse National Survey, 1995). Printed information about visual impairment and rehabilitation should be made available to older people to share with their families from the very start, preferably before the first contact—when a name and address are available to the agency. Not only does this approach signal the importance of family involvement and education, but it also leaves the educational process in the control of the older person—to distribute the material as he or she sees fit. For older people who are fearful of asking too much of their children or friends, this step also signals the appropriateness of reaching out to family members.

In this prerehabilitation phase, older people should be invited with family members to open houses or educational forums at the agency. Here, they can learn more about visual impairment and vision rehabilitation—all to the good for a successful launching of rehabilitation. In the group setting, the importance of appropriate family support can be emphasized. The Lighthouse International experience suggests that more informal open houses are less intimidating to older people and their families and that a convenient time and easily accessed location are important to ensure attendance. Whether taught in formal educational sessions or discussed in informal groups, the following subjects should be included:

1. A layperson's understanding of the major age-related vision diseases and conditions:

   ◆ The causes of age-related vision diseases and conditions, including genetic predisposition
   ◆ The potential and limitations of prevention and medical and surgical interventions
   ◆ Differentiation of diseases from normal age-related vision changes
   ◆ The impact of diseases on visual functioning
   ◆ The course of disease and functional changes over time

2. The components of vision rehabilitation

   ◆ Clinical low vision care, including assessment, prescription of devices, and training in their use
   ◆ Training in independent living techniques

3. The role of family members

   ◆ Support versus protection: doing too much; doing too little
   ◆ Understanding depressive reactions of the person with vision impairment

4. Stresses experienced by family members

Informal open houses and supportive educational programs for family members and older persons, given on a regular basis, should be a staple for any vision rehabilitation service before or after rehabilitation. There is little question that, armed with accurate information, some family members do not need additional services. They are well able to figure out on their own the appropriate role they can play. Others may require more assistance in understanding vision impairment and vision rehabilitation. Perhaps translated materials are required. Some may simply want to share experiences with other families. And, if the emotional and relational aspects related to the elderly relative's vision impairment are problematic, support groups or counseling may be required.

The type of family situation discerned in the assessment process or identified at a later time will determine whether to involve family members to a greater degree. If family members have participated in the assessment process and exhibit emotional or relational concern, family group sessions or support groups should be planned as a first order of business taking precedence over the sharing of information.

Support Groups

Families who are anxious or feel they are in crisis because of an older relative's vision impairment may both desire and benefit from support groups. Very often, spouses or other family members living in the same home may be particularly anxious and overprotective or feel burdened by the care they feel they must give or are required to give the older person. Both time-limited and continuing support groups for family members can be an effective means for the transmission of information about vision impairment and rehabilitation and for providing members emotional support. The sharing of concerns and emotional conflicts with persons in such situations can be very rewarding for some. The simple knowledge that one is not alone in a situation is supportive.

Care must be taken, however, that the older consumer does not feel excluded from these groups. In some situations, the isolation the older person is experiencing in relation to his family may only be reinforced if his or her spouse or child meet in separate groups. In other situations the separation can give some family members the distance they need to cope better. The timing of support group participation is important, as it was in the case of Mr. M. and his wife:

Mr. M., a 74-year-old retired government worker, lived with his wife of 35 years and near his three adult sons and their families. He had been very active in his community after retiring, but when he began to lose his vision as a result of macular degeneration, he became depressed and isolated and more dependent on his wife. His despair was so great that he demanded she leave her job. Mrs. M. was overwhelmed by her husband's demands on her, his emotional difficulties, and their growing marital conflicts. She took the lead in bringing a reluctant Mr. M. to the agency for a low vision examination.

The conflict between the couple was readily apparent when they appeared for the first visit, and the social worker engaged the couple in counseling for several visits to help them sort out their feelings and communicate more productively. Mr. M. became less resistive to rehabilitation and joined an adaptive skills training group. Regaining his confidence, he was able to give more support to his wife. She joined a spouse support group, which helped to reduce her anger. In time, Mr. M. was again active at home and in the community, and Mrs. M. had returned to her job.

Family Group Meetings

Family group meetings may be necessary for families in which constructive communication has broken down and there is a great deal of conflict in relation to the vision impairment. These sessions with the older client and family are held either in the home or at the agency. When the older person lives with a relative, these sessions may be interwoven with the skills training provided by the vision rehabilitation teacher in the home:

Mr. S., the spouse of 65-year-old Betty S., did not greet the rehabilitation specialist warmly when she made a home visit, in spite of his wife's eagerness to cook again. She had stopped doing most of her housework when her vision problem deteriorated further, as a result of diabetic retinopathy. The tension between her and her husband increased as he took over most of the household duties, to neither's satisfaction, and his overprotectiveness became, from her perspective, overbearing. He was very doubtful that his wife could benefit from vision rehabilitation. The therapist listened to his doubts, but persuaded the husband to observe the rehabilitation process so that he could understand the principles and techniques of adaptive skills training. Communication between the couple soon changed from a pattern of warnings, admonishments, and retorts to encouragement and support. Eventually, Mr. S. had time for himself again, and his resentment—which he had masked with domineering behavior—dissipated.

When family group sessions of this type are held in the agency with families who need a hands-on approach to understanding rehabilitation, the practice kitchen in the agency can be used or even a stroll outside practicing newly learned mobility skills. Rehabilitation therapists not trained in counseling can partner with a social worker or other type of family counselor for this type of work.

Group sessions are particularly appropriate for the family that is involved on a daily basis with the older person. Good communication that reflects support and interest is essential to a successful rehabilitation that otherwise can be sabotaged:

Ms. P., 61 years old, born and raised in Jamaica, lived with her 81-year-old mother and two granddaughters. She had lost her vision over 10 years ago and was cared for by her mother. Ms. P. was eager to travel independently again. Even though her mother accompanied Ms. P. to the agency, the mother vehemently opposed the rehabilitation plan, noting that caring for the family had always been her role. In several family meetings the social worker was able to help the daughter communicate her needs to her mother and to help the mother rethink her role in the family, while at the same time respecting the family's cultural background that strongly valued the mother's caregiving role. As the daughter acquired new skills in rehabilitation, both mother and daughter grew more confident and were able to do things independently of each other and share in household tasks.

There must be a *raison d'être* for gathering the family—not simply because it is the thing to do. The older person may request such a meeting to help in the process of alerting the family to the vision impairment or for asking for specific help. The worker may feel there is a lack of understanding of the vision impairment requiring more concentrated work with the family. Family group sessions should be initiated with clearly stated, agreed upon goals. In the case of Ms. P., the goal for the family meetings was to clarify and acknowledge the growing capabilities of Ms. P. and to make the necessary family adjustments that would foster these capabilities and in turn reduce the burden on other family members. As in the case of Ms. P., cultural factors that may influence the family's behavior must be factored not only into the assessment, but also into the dynamics of a family group meeting. Cultural factors were also significant for Mr. O. and his wife:

Mr. O., a 65-year-old retired Hispanic man, lived with his wife and four grandchildren. He and his wife cared for the children because of the mother's drug addiction. Mr. O. was visually impaired due to diabetic retinopathy and post-stroke complications. Mr. O.'s medical doctor referred him for vision rehabilitation services. At the first visit, Mr. O. appeared depressed and withdrawn, and there was a great deal of tension between him and his wife, who was overwhelmed by caring for him and the four grandchildren. Following the intake and assessment process, the social worker offered the couple the opportunity to discuss their problems with her. As an Hispanic person herself, she understood cultural taboos about "therapy" and exercised caution when engaging them in group counseling. After a few sessions, Mr. O. became more hopeful about his situation and moved ahead with a rehabilitation plan. At the same time, his wife felt more supported and, in turn, more supportive of him.

When the Family Is Not Involved

A family-oriented rehabilitation approach does not exclude those older clients whose families are not involved in rehabilitation.

Whether it is the family's choice to remain uninvolved or that of the older person, older consumers can profit from individual counseling and support groups that deal with their family situations. If they are alerted to the agency's family-oriented approach, they may spontaneously seek counseling in this area.

Mrs. K. was adamant that she did not want her children involved in her vision rehabilitation. She was fearful that if they knew about the extent of her vision problems, they would insist that she come live with them. Mrs. K. was eager to learn new skills so that she could demonstrate to them directly how well she could manage. The counselor helped her to see that the children might feel left out and hurt if they didn't know about her difficulties, thus creating a tense family situation. She helped Mrs. K. feel more confident about her ability to deal with her children and rehearse ways in which she could discuss her impairment with them now and walk them through the steps that would help her maintain her independence.

The key to persuading older consumers to involve their families is to help them understand that they can remain in control of their lives while at the same time seeking support from their families. This may not be possible until rehabilitation has progressed to the point that their confidence in themselves is restored. "Graduation" celebrations that mark the end of a phase of rehabilitation are an excellent means of involving family members previously on the periphery, as it was for Mrs. D.:

Mrs. D., a 61-year-old widow, was born with a high degree of myopia and struggled with vision problems from childhood. She married and raised four children independently after the death of her husband. Mrs. D. was recently diagnosed with glaucoma and suffered further vision loss which hampered her functioning. Her grown children, who lived

apart from her with their own families, had limited knowledge of her vision problem and, always having seen her as a
strong, independent woman, offered little support. For this
very reason, Mrs. D. refused to involve her children when
she came for rehabilitation services. The situation was complicated by the guilt Mrs. D. felt over the vision impairment
of one of her sons. As her adaptive skills training program
progressed, Mrs. D. became less depressed and more confident, and she invited her family to the graduation party. The
involvement of the family at this juncture helped them all to
see their avoidance of their mother's vision impairment and
address the fear for their own possible vision loss.

When the Family Is the Primary Client

If a family-oriented approach to vision rehabilitation for older people
is to be truly implemented, consideration should be given to offering
services to family members of an older, visually impaired relative who
is not involved in rehabilitation. This is the type of family situation in
which the family is alarmed about the poor vision of an older person
who is denying the problem. Outreach to these families can take place
through community forums, the media, and other community outlets.
A mechanism should be provided for family members to consult with
a member of the rehabilitation team. Their needs may be simple:
expert corroboration of their fears, which gives them the confidence to
speak with the older relative.

Perhaps the family has attempted to communicate with the older
person, but he or she refuses to acknowledge the problem or seek
help, even though his or her safety is compromised. This is a very
problematic situation involving deep fears on the part of the older
person, and such dysfunctional behavior usually negatively affects
other areas of his or her life as well. Referral of the family to a family
service agency or mental health clinic may be required.

BEYOND REHABILITATION

The feelings of family members about an older person's visual impairment must be placed in the larger context of the older person's life and

concerns for the future in general. It is the unusual family whose members are not also concerned about the occurrence of other age-related diseases and disabilities, so it behooves the rehabilitation agency to provide linkages for the older person and family to other providers in the aging network. It is also likely in the case of age-related vision loss that the underlying disease process will result in continuing deterioration of vision, requiring the services of a vision rehabilitation agency intermittently as the client ages.

Older persons and families should be encouraged to return for services if they are having difficulty with low vision devices or newly learned adaptive skills and when there is a change in vision functioning. If their concerns and anxieties are more pervasive, they should be referred to other community resources or support groups. The aging process itself and the increased risks for disability faced by older persons behooves the rehabilitation agency to alter its expectation of older clients. While there is little question that rehabilitation can help older visually impaired people enormously, the gains achieved can be lost without a long-term perspective for both older persons and families.

CONCLUSION

The family can be an important resource to the vision rehabilitation team in its work with older clients. Rather than being viewed as potential obstacles to rehabilitation, family members should be regarded as allies in the effort to maximize the elder's visual functioning and utilization of adaptive skills. With this perspective, concerned and anxious family members themselves feel supported and, for those who have filled a direct caregiving role, an unnecessary burden lifted as the older person is able to function more independently.

As recent experiences have shown, however, involving family members in the rehabilitation process is not a straightforward process. The needs of families vary widely depending on the impact of the elder's vision impairment on the lives of family members. Flexibility in programming and a long-term perspective are required. The differing degrees of readiness of older people to involve their families must be gauged and respected, and short-range rehabilitation goals placed within a long-term perspective.

REFERENCES

Antonucci, T. C. (1990). Social supports and social relationships. In R. H. Binstock & L. K. George (Eds.), *Handbook of aging and the social sciences* (pp. 205–226). San Diego, CA: Academic Press.

Administration on Aging. *Profile of older Americans: 1995.* (1996). Washington, DC: U.S. Department of Human Services.

Barer, B. M., & Johnson, C. L. (1990). A critique of the caregiving literature. *The Gerontologist, 30,* 26–29.

Bengtson, V. L., & Kuypers, J. (1971). Generational differences and the developmental stake. *Aging and Human Development, 2,* 249.

Branch, L. G., Horowitz, A., & Carr, C. (1989). The implications for everyday life of incident reported visual decline among people over age 65 living in the community. *The Gerontologist, 29,* 359–365.

Brody, E. M. (1985). Parent care as a normative family stress. *The Gerontologist, 25,* 19–29.

Brody, E. M. (1986). Informal support systems in the rehabilitation of the disabled elderly. In S. J. Brody & G. E. Ruff (Eds.), *Aging and rehabilitation: Advances in the state of the art* (pp. 87–103). New York: Springer.

Brody, S. J. & Ruff, G. E. (Eds.) (1986). *Aging and rehabilitation: Advances in the state of the art.* New York: Springer.

Cantor, M. H. (1983). Strain among caregivers: A study of experience in the United States. *The Gerontologist, 23,* 597–604.

Cantor, M., & Little, V. (1985). Aging and social care. In R. H. Binstock & E. Shanas (Eds.), *Handbook of aging and the social sciences* (2nd ed.). New York: Van Nostrand Reinhold.

Cicerelli, V. G. (1983). Adult children's attachment and helping behavior to elderly parents: A path model. *Journal of Marriage and the Family, 45,* 815–825.

Crews, J. E. (1991). Measuring rehabilitation outcomes and public policies of aging and blindness. In N. Miller (Ed.), *Vision and aging: Issues in social work practice.* New York: Haworth, pp. 137–151.

Crews, J. E., & Frey, W. D. (1993). Family concerns and older people who are blind. *Journal of Visual Impairment & Blindness, 87* (1), 6–11.

Evans, R. L., Bishop, D. S., & Haselkorn, J. K. (1991). Factors predicting satisfactory home care after stroke. *Archives of Physical Medicine and Rehabilitation, 72,* 144–147.

Greenblatt, S. L. (1988). Physicians and chronic impairment: A study of ophthalmologists' interactions with visually impaired and blind patients. *Social Science Medicine, 26,* 393–399.

Grieg, D. E., West, M. I., & Overbury, O. (1986). Successful use of low vision aids: Visual and psychological factors. *Journal of Visual Impairment & Blindness, 80* (10), 985–988.

Hersen, M., Kabacoff, R. I., Van Hasselt, U. B., Null, J. A., Ryan, C. F., Melton, M. A., & Segal, D. L. (1995). Assertiveness, depression, and social support in older visually impaired adults. *Journal of Visual Impairment & Blindness, 89* (6), 524–530.

Hofland, B. (1988). Autonomy in long term care: Background issues and a programmatic response. *The Gerontologist, 28* (Suppl.) 3–9.

Horowitz, A. (1985). Family caregiving to the frail elderly. In M. P. Lawton & G. Maddox (Eds.), *The annual review of gerontology and geriatrics.* New York: Springer, pp. 194–246.

Horowitz, A., Bird, B., Goodman, C. R., Reinhardt, J. P., Flynn, M. A., Silverstone, B., & Cantor, M. (1998). *Vision rehabilitation and family services: Maximizing functional and psychosocial status for both older visually impaired adults and their families.* Final Report. New York: The Lighthouse Inc.

Horowitz, A. & Reinhardt, J. R. (1992). *Assessing adaptation to age-related vision loss.* New York: The Lighthouse Research Institute.

Horowitz, A., Silverstone, B., & Reinhardt, J. (1991). A conceptual and empirical exploration of personal autonomy issues within family caregiving relationships. *The Gerontologist, 31,* 23–31.

Kaufman, R., Albright, L., & Wagner, C. (1987). Rehabilitation outcomes after hip fracture in persons 90 years old and older. *Archives of Physical and Medical Rehabilitation, 68,* 369–371.

Kemp, B. (1986). Psychosocial and mental health issues in rehabilitation of older persons. In S. J. Brody & G. E. Ruff (Eds.) *Aging and rehabilitation: Advances in the state of the art.* New York: Springer, pp. 122–58.

Kemp, B., Brummel-Smith, K., & Ramsdell, J. W. (Eds.) (1990). *Geriatric Rehabilitation.* Boston, MA: College-Hill Press.

Large, T. (1982). Effects of attitudes upon the blind: A re-examination. *Journal of Rehabilitation, 48,* 33–34, 45.

Lidoff, L. (1997). Moving vision-related rehabilitation into the U.S. Health care mainstream. *Journal of Vision Impairment & Blindness, 91*(2), 107–116.

The Lighthouse national survey on vision loss: The experience, attitudes and knowledge of middle-aged and older Americans. (1995). New York: The Lighthouse Inc., Arlene R. Gordon Research Institute.

McNett, S. C. (1987). Social support, threat and coping responses and effectiveness in the functionally disabled. *Nursing Research, 36,* 98–103.

Oakes, T. W., Ward, J. R., Grey, R. M., et al. (1970). Family expectation and arthritis patient compliance to a hand resting splint regimen. *Journal of Chronic Diseases, 22,* 757–764.

Oppegard, K., Hansson, R. O., Morgan, T., et al. (1984). Sensory loss, family support, and adjustment among the elderly. *The Journal of Social Psychology, 123,* 291–292.

Rabins, P. V., Mace, N. L., & Lucas, M. J. (1982). The impact of dementia on the family. *Journal of the American Medical Association, 248,* 333–335.

Reece, D., Walz, T., & Hageboeck, H. (1983). Intergenerational care providers of non-institutionalized frail elderly: Characteristics and consequences. *Journal of Gerontological Social Work, 15,* 21–34.

Reinhardt, J. P. (1996). The importance of friendship and family support in adaptation to chronic vision impairment. *Journal of Gerontology: Psychological Sciences, 51b,* 268–278.

Rogers, P., & Long, R. G. (1991). The challenge of establishing a national service delivery program for older blind adults. In N. Miller (Ed.), *Vision and aging: Issues in social work practice.* New York: Haworth, pp. 137–151.

Shanas, E. (1979). The family as a social support system in old age. *The Gerontologist, 19,* 169–174.

Shenkel, R., Rogers, J., Perfeito, G. & Levin, R. (1985–86). Importance of "significant others" in predicting cooperation with diabetic regression. *Journal of Psychiatry in Medicine, 15,* 149–155.

Silverstone, B. (1985). Informal support systems for the frail elderly. In *America's Aging: Health in an older society.* Washington, DC: Institute of Medicine and National Research Council, National Academy Press.

Silverstone, B. (1993). Beyond the boundaries of normal aging: The case of age related vision loss. *The Gerontologist, 33* (4), 566–567.

Thomas, T., & Stevens, R. (1974). Social effects of fractures of the femur. *British Medical Journal, 3,* 456–458.

Weinberger, M. (1980). Social and psychological consequences of legitimating a hearing impairment. *Social Science Medicine, 14,* 213–222.

Williams, T. F. (Ed.) (1984). *Rehabilitation in the aging.* New York: Raven Press.

CHAPTER 8

Aging and Disabilities: Collaborative Practice and Public Policy

Edward F. Ansello

The survival to later life of persons with formerly life-stunting disabilities has been one of the significant achievements of the late twentieth century. It has been made possible by several factors, including life-sustaining interventions in pharmacology, which often prevent mid-life impairments that occur on top of lifelong disabilities from proving fatal, and the increased life expectancies of family caregivers, most often the parents of the persons with disabilities, enabling them to continue their care for a longer period of time. The achievement of this survival to later life, however, has been presented to a society largely unprepared to accept the gift. Examination of practice and policy responses to the aging of persons with lifelong, developmental disabilities may be instructive for suggesting initiatives related to aging and visual impairment.

EVOLUTIONS IN AGING AND DISABILITY

Our society has been facing two evolutions in this era: the aging of the nation as a whole and the increasing longevity of persons with serious disabilities. With regard to the former, it can be argued that such social institutions as the family, work life, education, and government have reacted to, but have not fully integrated, the implications of much longer human life expectancy. The creation of new life stages, such as prolonged adolescence, young adulthood, and gradations of later life, are redefining family life. Prolonged physical and intellectual vigor are compelling ongoing reassessments of job commitments, employer–employee relationships, and the age of retirement. Women now complete traditional child-rearing responsibilities at a point in life at which on average they can expect more years ahead than they had previously lived as an adult. As a result, women are transforming the landscape of higher education and are "feminizing" previously male-dominated occupations for which that education prepares them, including medicine and business. The wide broadcast of the gift of time—that is, the benefits of longevity reaching people irrespective of gender, race, socioeconomic status, or physical history—has meant continuous reappraisal by all levels of government of entitlement programs and safety nets, and of the very role of government itself, because government support (e.g., Social Security and Medicaid) will spread over a much longer potential time-frame than ever before.

The evolution of disability can be expected to produce an even greater lack of preparedness in social institutions than that which characterized the awakening to an aging America in the 1970s and 1980s. In a United States in which not only average citizens live much longer than before but also those with disabilities enjoy fuller life expectancies, formal, bureaucratic systems will be challenged to respond. And because the response of social institutions is typically slow, many of those affected will not wait but will attempt to foment change. Moreover, in a culture in which independence and assertiveness are valued, those first to speak out, to coalesce, and to advocate tend to gather the greatest attention and social response.

Since the aging of the nation struck public consciousness first, aging-related concerns have been more prominent in popular culture (e.g., the media) than those that are disabilities related, and aging-related advocacy groups tend to be more powerful politically than disabilities groups. The common experience of growing older broadens the clout of aging advocates in ways that the disabilities community may never achieve. At the same time, while it is inherently contrary to logic, few people aspire to be old. Aging remains a begrudged denouement of a life of prolonged youthfulness. In short, aging is a marginalized value. Like the margin of a page, aging is on the border or at the edge of the socially valued text that tells stories of productivity, independence, and attractiveness.

From this brief appraisal we can abstract some current realities vis-à-vis public policy and practice related to aging and disabilities:

1. The field of aging is more established and perceived to be more politically cohesive than is the disabilities field.
2. Although somewhat more socially acceptable, aging shares with disabilities a marginalized status.
3. Advocacy groups within each area, that is, aging and disabilities, may serve both to shed light upon common issues and to fragment the focus of public attention.
4. Some social institutions are more advanced than others in their response to the broad developments in aging and disabilities and to their particular consequences. Families, for instance, have proven remarkably flexible and adaptive. They endure, having incorporated such aging-related attributes as multiple generations, empty nest renaissance, and extended retirement, as well as other attributes characteristic of both aging and disabilities, such as family caregiving and planning for children to outlive parents. Other social institutions, such as government and organized religion, have been less responsive to these aging-and disabilities-driven concerns. Families, therefore, may be a productive focal point for initiatives on aging and disabilities, including aging and vision loss.

The separate evolutions of the fields of aging and of disabilities and their parallel universes intersect where persons with disabilities grow older. The aging of large numbers of individuals with lifelong impairments has drawn the two "systems" into contact with each other. For the past decade or so, researchers, educators, practitioners, managers, policymakers, and others in the aging network and in the disabilities system have mingled episodically. They have explored their similarities and differences in priorities, funding streams, services, and training. Model projects have initiated collaborations in client outreach, cross-training, and resource sharing. Some realities emerge from a distillation of these experiences.

WHY COLLABORATE?

Experiences driven by the aging of persons with lifelong disabilities[1] may well be instructive for those working at the intersection of aging and visual rehabilitation. Older persons with lifelong disabilities are pulling the aging and developmental disabilities systems into the intersection. Not every contact results in cooperation, however, let alone formal programs such as the several Partners Projects with which the author was associated (Ansello, Coogle, & Wood, 1997; Ansello, Wells, & Zink, 1989; Coogle, Ansello, Wood, & Cotter, 1995; Cotter, Ansello, & Wood, 1992) and other government-supported initiatives. The Partners Projects were a series of initiatives funded by the Administration on Aging from 1987 through 1996 that sought to identify the prevalence, characteristics, and needs of older adults in the community with developmental disabilities, and to help establish cooperation between the aging and developmental disabilities service systems to benefit these adults and their families. A necessary precondition for intersystem cooperation seems to be a general awareness of the benefits, both immediate and long-term. These might include a broader range of options for the individual, the planner, and the provider; joint case management; avoidance of duplicative services; cost-effective resource sharing; reciprocal (and often no-cost) cross-training; evidence

---

[1]Both the terms *disability* and *developmental disability* are used throughout this chapter. The latter has a more restrictive denotation, referring to a severe, chronic disability with an early onset that results in substantial functional limitations and is likely to continue indefinitely. Because of the mix of studies and projects referenced here, practice and policy implications are generally assumed to apply to both disabilities and developmental disabilities systems. When findings derive only from projects on developmental disabilities, this is so noted.

of support for agencies' budget appropriations; and preparation and skills development for future needs, benefitting consumers, caregivers, planners, and providers.

In addition to awareness of these benefits, local units in the two fields and their state-level directorates need to anticipate some proximate benefits to themselves of intersystem cooperation. Experience suggests that this expectation moves intersystem cooperation from a concept to an action. A nationwide survey of state-level aging and developmental disabilities units undertaken to identify the "hot-button issues" they are dealing with vis-à-vis aging with lifelong disabilities found that for many the issue is a non-issue (Coogle, Ansello, Wood, & Cotter, 1997). The small numbers of elders with developmental disabilities, estimated at 1 percent of the population age 60 years and above (Ansello & Eustis, 1992), was justifying their doing little or nothing. These national findings support an earlier assessment of 13 agencies in Virginia that were responsible for older people with various developmental disabilities; this survey found that a passive and reactive rather than an active philosophy was typical of agencies' efforts in identifying clients, allocating resources, funding, and providing services for the specific population of older persons with developmental disabilities (Coogle, Ansello, Wood, & Cotter, 1995).

The current state of services targeted to older persons with developmental disabilities, therefore, tends to be passive, with individual agencies responding to requests and referrals, rather than initiating or coordinating actions. Implementing intersystem or even intrasystem cooperation represents a significant increase in initiative. The impetus for this initiative may come from any of several sources—caregivers, advocates, bureaucrats, service providers, elected officials, planners, and others. One group, one subset within a group, or even one person can create the spark and lead the way to cooperation. The catalyst, however, remains anticipating practical benefits from collaboration.

Elements within each system have begun explorations with counterparts in the other. These explorations have revealed a number of instructive observations about the relationships between the fields that are pertinent in considering collaborations between the aging and developmental disabilities fields. It seems reasonable to assume that these principles will be relevant as well to the fields of vision rehabilitation and late-onset disabilities such as Alzheimer's disease, Parkinson's disease, and stroke. These observations are as follows:

1. The fields of aging and disabilities share a marginal status in society.
2. The process of advocacy by one group frequently clouds the similarities it has with the other.
3. Chronic care by families is a value common to the fields of both aging and disability.
4. The field of aging is being medicalized, and self-care is being challenged.
5. Alliances and coalitions between the fields of aging and disabilities are inherently unfavorable to the strong and more helpful to the weak members.
6. The thrust in both aging and disabilities is toward more and more local arenas of operation.
7. Models of collaboration between aging and disabilities have been tested and may be applied.

These observations are discussed in detail in the sections that follow.

A COMMON MARGINALIZATION

The fields of aging and disabilities share a marginal status in society. Elders and those with disabilities, whether lifelong, late-onset, or otherwise, share a marginalized status. They may be objectified, negatively evaluated against some standard of productivity, imputed to be suffering (and in need of release), and compartmentalized outside of the average person's concern. These unfortunate circumstances owe much to our response to these persons rather than to the intrinsic impairments they may have. Zola (1988) reminds us that "disabling conditions are not merely the result of some physical or mental impairment, but rather of the fit of such impairments with the social, attitudinal, architectural, and even political environment" (p. 369).

The aged and those with disabilities share similar assessments in Callahan's (1987) thoughtful treatment on the demands being placed upon medicine, medical technology, and the social economics that fuel them. In *Setting Limits* he concludes that certain classes of people, including the aged, newborns with congenital impairments, and people with serious disabilities, have needs that exceed reasonable care. Addressing their conditions would exhaust resources and would thereby benefit the few at the expense of the many. At the root of Callahan's argument is an unstated objectification of these groups. They are presumed to be unproductive or never-to-be productive members of the society.

In a lineage stretching at least from the eugenics movement of the 1880s to the 1940s through current debates over euthanasia, some ethicists have argued the premise that another's existence can be objectified and evaluated; that is, value can be measured rationally against some calibrated standard, such as economic productivity, either current or projected, or contributions to societal well-being. In these evaluations, those with disabilities and those with infirmities of age, or, at times, simply advanced age itself, have fared poorly. Pernick (1996) and Goldhagen (1996), respectively, cite examples of active and passive euthanasia of babies diagnosed as "defective" early in this century and statewide elimination of individuals classified as "defectives" by the Nazi regime in Germany. Ethicists justified these interventions on the grounds of the individual's nonproductivity, unreasonable consumption of medical and economic resources, or "suffering." Presence of a disability was equated with suffering, and eliminating the suffering justified the intervention or nonintervention, as the case might dictate. Of course, those objectified were not necessarily asked about their presumed suffering. Differing perceptions between physicians and adults, both young and old, regarding the relative benefits and burdens of such life-sustaining interventions as artificial nutrition and hydration and cardiopulmonary resuscitation, where physicians rate the benefits lower and the burdens higher, may reflect a residual of this ethic (Coppola, Danks, Ditto, & Smucker, 1998).

Today, the more enlightened community recognizes that societal exclusions or restrictions, as much as the disabilities themselves, contribute to inferior quality of life and suffering. These conditions are remediable; the individuals need not be expendable. Nonetheless, elders and individuals with disabilities often share the designation of "suffering," as in "suffering from cerebral palsy" or "suffering from old age." At the extreme, some would relieve suffering through euthanasia; more moderately, many separate from their own everyday world those whom they objectify as suffering. The latter cause discomfort; they cost rather than contribute; they are marginalized.

Not incidentally, one of the earliest countermeasures undertaken to this marginalization was to institute training programs to make those with disabilities more fit for employment. Vocational training or rehabilitation promised to create productive and contributing citizens. In short, work would set marginalized people free of negative evaluations. When trained for an occupation, they would become contributing members of society. Vocational rehabilitation programs were developed for individuals who were blind and visually impaired. Agencies serving people with mental retardation or developmental disabilities employed similar vocational training schemes, legitimizing appropriations through job training, even when a lifetime of training might fail to prepare some individuals for work because of the severity of their disabilities, and even when an organization's philosophical commitment to job training might preclude an individual's ever retiring from that training.

Consistent with the ethic of overcoming marginalization through productivity, or at least through job training for productivity, training for older blind and visually impaired persons that was not related to employment failed to receive appropriations for many years, and training for retirement from job training for older adults with mental retardation has only lately begun to appear in the curricula that prepare professionals for the developmental disabilities field (Sterns, Heller, Sterns, Factor, & Miklos, 1994; Sterns, Kennedy-Hart, Sed, & Heller, in press). In the former instance, Title VII, Part C of the Rehabilitation Act of 1973, which aimed to ensure that training for independent living for older blind persons was not tied to their employability, was authorized in the original legislation but failed to receive appropriations for more than a dozen years. In the latter instance, while there are many organizational variations within the states, the funding stream for mental retardation or developmental disability is essentially one where "the money follows the individual," so an elder's withdrawal from a job training "slot" has often been thought to jeopardize funding of that site.

Becoming aware that the people they care for share societal marginalization, those committed to the aging and disabilities fields can use this commonality to undertake activities that share common ideals, perhaps use shared resources, and produce results of mutual benefit. The first step in collaborative practice and policy development is overcoming the "us" versus "them" syndrome.

COMMON ISSUES

The process of advocacy by one group frequently clouds the similarities it has with the other groups. However, with the equanimity of one contemplating a half-filled or half-empty glass of water, it is possible to declare that the aging and disabilities fields, confronting the aging of persons with disabilities (either developmental or late-onset), have more in common than in contrast. It is immediately acknowledged that the term "fields" is comfortably loose. The aging network is a hierarchical stream for funds to flow from the federal Administration on Aging to State Units on Aging and on to Area Agencies on Aging in order to benefit the largest number of persons who are entitled to services by virtue of chronological age.

The developmental disabilities system is far more fragmented, with mental retardation enjoying the dominant position among these disabilities for obtaining resources, by virtue of its stronger history of grassroots advocacy, organizational sophistication, and professional development. Persons with developmental disabilities often receive the services they need to maximize their potential level of functioning, but they are selected rather than entitled, and waiting lists for services are common. Moreover, because of the identification of developmental disabilities with mental retardation, some advocates and organizations for people with other lifelong developmental disabilities choose not to associate themselves with the label of developmental disabilities, even when the consumers they serve have conditions that meet the functional definitions of a developmental disability. This is defined by PL 95–602 and PL 101–496, the Developmental Disabilities Act and Bill of Rights, as a severe, chronic disability, attributable to a mental or physical impairment or a combination of both, that manifests before age 22, which is likely to continue indefinitely, results in at least three substantial functional limitations, and requires a combination of extended or lifelong services. Because this definition is functional rather than categorical, developmental disabilities may include mental retardation, cerebral palsy, autism, blindness, deafness, orthopedic disabilities, multiple disabilities, and other lifelong disabilities. Yet, in many instances, advocates and organizations from these other developmental disabilities elect not to enter coalitions or partnerships, not to stand under the developmental disabilities umbrella, because it is being held by mental retardation. They choose to highlight their differences rather than their similarities.

Notwithstanding these fundamental differences, the aging and disabilities fields share a number of common issues. Recognizing these similarities may facilitate intermural and intramural cooperation that benefits aging persons with disabilities. Issues that cut across both fields include the importance of consumers assuming more responsibility for their own services, the heterogeneity of the consumer population, and the need for greater clarity about the goals of the field.

Contributions by Consumers

Elders and persons with disabilities tend unfairly to be seen only as recipients of services rather than as agents of these services. Both the aging and disabilities fields are beginning to recognize that many times their consumers do not wish to be passive recipients but rather seek to be active players in their own care or in the provision of services to others. Senior centers that are inundated administratively with a ratio of 400 to 500 members to one full-time paid staff person find relief, and organizational growth, when elderly members assume more responsibility for management, programming, outreach, etc. In the evolution of adult care centers in the aging field, and of personal care services in both the aging and developmental disabilities systems, consumers seek more control over the services they receive, demanding the right to hire, train, supervise, and fire those who provide services to them. In one situation the power and sensitivity of caring were evident in an exchange between two "clients," an older adult with Down syndrome who was carefully feeding an elder with Alzheimer's disease, while both attended an adult day care center.

Heterogeneity

The dynamic of human development increases differentiation within a group as its members grow older. Simply put, humans grow less and less like each other as they age (Ansello & Eustis, 1992; Ansello & Rose, 1989). This imperative is not abrogated because of the presence of disabilities, whether lifelong or late-onset. Those who work with mainstream adults who acquire disabilities late in life or adults who grow old with developmental disabilities face in common a group that is growing more heterogeneous. Their diversity in attitude, functional capacity, philosophical outlook, spiritual grounding, economic wherewithal, behavior, informal supports, and much more stamps each person as an individual, challenging if not frustrating uniform, categorical responses to them. Individuals with the same diagnosis will require more or less assistance, need more or less direction, and assume more or less responsibility, with more or less humor than others. Partnerships across and within the systems bring resources. Recognizing that consumers, in common, are growing more heterogeneous, practitioners may borrow strategies from each other that have proven to be effective.

Clarity of Goals

Both the aging and disabilities fields have responded to the evolution within their consumer bases with episodes of energy between periods of confusion. As the number of mainstream elders swelled since passage of the Older Americans Act of 1965, their emerging needs and capacities dictated first one then another priority for appropriations. Consider the assigned function over the years of the senior center: congregate meals and nutrition site, social-recreational outlet, community focal point, provider of social or medical adult day care, and so on. Similarly, as adults with developmental disabilities age, some within the developmental disability system question whether these individuals should continue the job training that may have defined their lives and the agency's function. As these individuals age, should they use existing "generic" senior services in the broader community, or should the developmental disabilities system develop its own age-segregated programs? More basically, as adults with lifelong disabilities grow old, are they the responsibility of the disabilities system or the aging system? The question is clouded further by the acquisition of late-onset disabilities such as post-stroke aphasia or Alzheimer's disease on top of lifelong, developmental disabilities.

The intersection of the aging and disabilities systems brought about by the aging of those with disabilities and the disabling of those with age offers an opportunity to sort out the most appropriate goals for each system so that those it serves may benefit. Interaction is likely to reveal that an either/or mentality regarding where "clients" belong or who provides services is short sighted.

ROLE OF THE FAMILY

Chronic care by families is a value common to the fields of both aging and disabilities. One of the most fundamental issues common to both the aging and disabilities fields is the central role that the family plays in chronic caregiving. Families have provided both the initial and the sustaining care that has maintained today's elders with lifelong disabilities in the community. Before federal mainstreaming education legislation was passed in the 1960s and 1970s (culminating in the Education for All Handicapped Children Act of 1975 and the later Individuals with Disabilities Education Act), interventions that help mark young adult and early middle-aged adults with developmental disabilities as more self-care-oriented than their aging counterparts, families provided the care necessary to keep their sons and daughters in the community. They continue this care to their aging children today. In parallel, when late-onset disabilities occur, daughters and wives are most likely to assume responsibility for chronic care. Far from institutionalizing older people with disabilities, extraordinary measures are taken to keep them within the community.

A 1988 study of caregivers of persons with need for assistance in two or more instrumental activities of daily living or one activity of daily living (ADL) found some seven million caregiving households in the United States (American Association for Retired Persons & The Travelers Foundation, 1988). When these criteria were applied in 1996, the number of caregiving households had tripled, to over 21 million (National Alliance for Caregiving & American Association of Retired Persons, 1997). The latter study identified approximately three-quarters of the care recipients as being 50 years of age or older. Doty, Jackson, and Crown (1998), using data from the 1989 National Long-Term Care Survey and the Informal Caregivers Survey, report that almost half of the primary caregivers of elders with disabilities are themselves aged 65 or older. They found, moreover, that employed female caregivers for elders with severe disabilities (three to five ADL impairments) still manage to provide between 32 and 39 hours of care a week. These caregivers tend to maintain high levels of care while employed by sharing residence with the care recipient, either in the elder's or the caregiver's home.

The U.S. General Accounting Office (1998) reports that spending for long-term care for the elderly totaled almost $91 billion in 1995, the most recent year for complete data; almost 40 percent of these monies were provided by the elders and their families. The Congressional Budget Office notes that, in national health expenditures between 1980 and 1990, that portion paid by private sources increased more than did either the federal portion or the state and local government portion (Anonymous, 1998). Nor should the value of family caregiving be limited to dollars. Examining the costs of care for dementia incurred by families, Strommel, Collins, and Given (1994) found that cash expenditures account for only 29 percent of total costs, with unpaid labor by the families making up the difference. Time is money, but time tends not to be calculated in the costs that are associated with chronic care.

Family caregiving is a vital, under-recognized element of the long-term care system, as well as being a common undergirding of both the aging and disabilities fields. Families provide both the money and the time required to maintain older adults with disabilities in the community. In many ways, this assistance from families lessens the load on institutions of care and on service systems such as the aging and disabilities fields. Family caregiving may postpone entry to nursing homes for persons with Alzheimer's disease. When caregivers receive comprehensive support and counseling, institutionalization may be postponed almost a year beyond the entry time where caregivers receive no such assistance (Mittelman, Ferris, Schulman, Steinberg, & Levin, 1996). Similarly, demand for more intensive levels of care within the developmental disabilities system may be lessened through recognition of the central role that families play in maintaining chronic care and reinforcement of their capacities.

With no major increase in funding for aging network and developmental disabilities services on the horizon, it seems prudent and practical for these systems to work together to strengthen the abilities of family caregivers to continue their care. The several Partners Projects found that family caregivers wanted to know more about existing community resources so that they could continue to do what they were doing, that is, providing chronic care to aging family members with lifelong disabilities (Ansello et al., 1997; Cotter et al., 1992). Far from adding to the agency's caseloads, the projects' outreach to family caregivers demonstrated that families are interested in practical training and information that would sustain their *non-use* of the agency's services. Family caregivers seek information on existing resources in the community for respite, networking with other caregivers and the rest of the community, receiving reliable information on Social Security and Medicare, and, to a lesser extent, planning for the continued care of their family member after the caregivers' death (Ansello et al., 1997). Family caregivers of aging adults with developmental disabilities seem so externally focused on the recipient of their care that they appear to postpone indefinitely their own mid-life confrontation with aging and mortality. Instead, these caregivers assume that they will maintain a level of energy characteristic of their earlier years and continue the daily routine to maintain normalcy for the care recipient. They often deny focus on themselves and fail to plan for the continued care of the recipient after their own demise.

MEDICALIZATION OF AGING

The field of aging is being medicalized and self-care is being challenged. Specifically, both academic gerontology and formal caregiving services for elders are increasingly becoming medicalized. Centers on aging, gerontology programs and departments, and other aging-related units in academe are in transition, with physicians being appointed to chairs in both newly developed and established settings. Although this may signal a greater level of commitment to the programs by the academic administration and may convey an elevated status for the program in the eyes of some, gerontological research and training emphases that are socioeconomic, affective, behavioral, recreational, or otherwise nonclinical become supplanted by emphases on biomedical, physiological, or pharmacological issues. As important as the latter emphases are, the effect, at times, is to transform the aging person or the person with disabilities into a patient.

Less precipitously but as pervasively, aging-related services have become medicalized. The evolution of the senior center's purposes, mentioned earlier, has not been haphazard but directional, toward serving the more frail, more impaired elder. Thus, senior centers have created adjunctive adult daycare centers, and provision of already stretched services is more often by triage, with the most vulnerable individuals having first claim. This shift in focus toward a more medicalized model for aging-related research, training, and service has occurred with less disruption than might otherwise be expected because of a prevailing ethic that can be described as paternalistic. The aging network has historically been management and staff driven.

Input from consumers mattered little when numbers served as the funding criterion.

The medicalization of the aging network and, more broadly, of the field of aging has untoward consequences, however, for the nascent self-care movement within the field, as well as for partnerships or coalitions with the developmental disabilities field where client-centered and client-directed services are the paradigm given the greatest lip service, if not the most active endorsement. Nor is a bridge readily constructed between the two fields without first acknowledging the degrees of control guarded by many agencies and professionals in human service. As Gilson and Netting (1997) observe in an essay for social workers,

> Commonly, agencies that are designated service providers for disabled people and for people who are aging have structural and organizational policies and procedures that not only block the practice of self-determination, but actively discourage it. The social worker then may be faced with helping the individual develop a belief in his or her capacity to self-determine the services needed, as well as working to change the agency practices that run counter to consumer-defined and consumer-directed services. Practicing self-determination, the choice and direction of one's goods and services requires just that: practice. Because people often hold paternalistic attitudes toward disabled and elderly people, these two groups of individuals have been discouraged from practicing true choice and self-direction. For agencies, this simply means working to individualize services to fit the individual, rather than fit the individual to the available services. (p. 296)

Recently in Virginia, certain state agencies proposed expanding the personal assistance services program to cover more aged clients. Client self-direction is at the core of the personal assistance services program. Although aging and disabilities advocates were not diametrically opposed to each other's positions, and the majority favored the expansion, the aging field accounted for the most outspoken opponents of personal assistance services for elders.

Family caregiving, acknowledged as key by both fields, is not antithetical to self-care. While adults with disabilities themselves disagree (frequently along generational lines) on the primacy of self-care versus family caregiving in continued community living, emphasizing either self-care or family caregiving involves a recognition of the individual as a person, not as a patient, and actualizes the role of agency staff as assistants to care outside the agency.

The provision of assistive devices may underscore the shared goal of both self-care and family caregiving, namely, enhancing the continuation of relatively independent living in the community. Assistive devices tend to be designed not for a given age but rather for a given condition. Low vision magnifiers are of equal assistance to the caregiving parent as to the aging son with a developmental disability when vision is impaired. Tear-away clothing, built-up utensils, enlarged numbers on the telephones and clocks, medication management aids, adapted bathroom fixtures, and chairs that assist one in rising are all similarly relevant to persons identified as participants in either the aging system or the developmental disabilities system, when enhancing functioning is the goal.

BENEFITS OF COALITIONS

Alliances and coalitions between the fields of aging and disabilites are mutually beneficial to the strong and to the weak members. As noted elsewhere (Ansello et al., 1997), aging and developmental disability service systems must collaborate in order to support independent living and prevent inappropriate institutionalization for persons who are aging and have disabilities. The field of aging has had little experience with disabilities, and little experience with individually tailored services. The disabilities field, especially developmental disabilities, has had little experience with aging. Until recently, few persons with developmental disabilities survived to late life, so interventions and the funding that accompanies them were targeted to early life, in the hope of improving the course of life.

Partnering across the fields and within the disabilities can generate adequate planning and improved service availability, so that older persons with developmental disabilities may be able to participate in and contribute to community life, receive appropriate services, and maintain their desired lifestyle. Collaboration makes these outcomes more likely, but collaboration begs a purpose, an ultimate goal, for the collaboration and requires certain principles of operation in working together toward attaining the goal. Agreeing to a common goal for all participants in a collaboration is the essential, nonmodifiable first step. Unless all parties agree and the organizations they represent substantiate that agreement by actions, such as memoranda of agreement or of commitment to the process, partnerships soon devolve into meetings for other agenda. In setting goals and in working toward achieving them, each participant in a coalition must carry equal weight. The largest and the smallest organizations in a partnership each must have one vote; otherwise, the dominance that exists outside the collaboration is reproduced.

Participants in an alliance work toward achieving goals of mutual benefit. Enlightened self-interest may be a motivator, but always with a view toward improving or maintaining the status of the consumer. This democracy tends to benefit weaker or smaller organizations more than larger, for each has not only equal voting or input but also access to some aspect of the other's resources, and, of course, larger organizations have more resources to be accessed. Although smaller organizations tend to benefit disproportionately, the impetus for the alliance is to grow beyond current levels of achievement, so all participants gain from alliance.

Coalitions between organizations involved in aging and disabilities in our experiences have a number of goals of mutual benefit to their members. These goals have included the following:

◆ *Cross-training of their staff on topics related to aging with disabilities.* The training is invariably provided without cost by fellow members of the coalition, and again smaller organizations gain access to the depth and breadth of training expertise of the other coalition members.

◆ *Support for caregivers.* This may entail offering training programs and workshops on such issues as nutrition and well-being for caregivers, permanency planning, medication management, and advocacy, as well as holding resource fairs to showcase the variety of resources available in the community, from state and local governmental to for-profit and non-profit.

◆ *Adapted design.* Both aging and disabilities participants have an interest in helping consumers to make full use of assistive devices. "Gadgets and Gizmos" fairs have been especially well received for effectively demonstrating the range of low-tech to high-tech devices that enable some degree of self-sufficiency or ease of care.

◆ *Public awareness.* Coalitions have developed campaigns to educate the public about the realities of aging with disabilities, the need of individuals with disabilities for community inclusion and opportunities to contribute, the gap between needs and resources, the primacy of family caregiving, and the life course of certain disabilities (e.g., post-polio syndrome).

Less successfully, coalitions have tried to establish single points of access whereby older adults with disabilities may enter the human services network only once, perhaps by completing a comprehensive assessment whose results are shared among pertinent agencies. Progress toward the goal of creating service credit banking operations in communities has been equally slow. These banks function like cooperatives where services to members are provided by members and credited against future need. Supported by the Robert Wood Johnson Foundation and administered by the University of Maryland Center on Aging, the service credit banking project had banks operational or planned in 29 states as of January 1997. The project provides start-up technical assistance and publishes a newsletter on volunteer credit exchange.

Experience has also suggested that the more creative the alliance, the more innovative the likely outcomes. Hence, the Partners Projects have encouraged local and statewide coalitions composed of consumers and family caregivers, plus representatives from the field of aging, advocates for the several developmental disabilities, adult protective services, parks and recreation, public health, and mental health. Some alliances also have included agency representatives and advocates for late-onset disabilities, such as Alzheimer's disease,

Parkinson's disease, stroke, and heart disease. Conceptually, the alliances create a triangle, with aging, lifelong disabilities, and late-onset disabilities occupying each of the angles and articulation between adjoining sectors taking place along each of the sides. In practice, many of the participants from these three sectors share such common needs as improving resource utilization, complementing existing resources, augmenting staff development, justifying budget requests, increasing public awareness, and so forth. Recently, a small number of partnerships have begun to explore inviting prevention-oriented groups into the alliance, groups such as Mothers Against Drunk Driving and those that target crime prevention. The motivation is recognition that improvements in medical intervention and technology increasingly mean that younger persons injured traumatically by drunk driving accidents or criminal violence are likely to survive the trauma to live the rest of their lives with disabilities. Thus, these horrific events are factories producing adults who grow old with disabilities.

As hopeful as these creative alliances are, those between academics and practitioners in the aging and developmental disabilities fields are equally promising. Notwithstanding the insinuation of medicalization into academic gerontology, a number of innovative model projects have been supported by the U.S. Administration on Aging or the Administration on Developmental Disabilities. Four projects supported by the Administration on Aging are illustrative. Clark and Susa (in press) of the University of Rhode Island conducted the Family Futures Training Project in that state. Using a carefully developed and tested educational intervention, they assisted family caregivers to identify and move beyond barriers that had prevented them from instituting permanency planning for the continuing care of their family members with developmental disabilities. Collaboration among family members, consumers, and agency staffs from the aging and disabilities fields was key to success of the project. Factor (1996) and colleagues at the University of Illinois at Chicago established coalitions in rural, inner-city Hispanic, and suburban locations to improve outreach to at-risk families, encourage families to make future plans to avert crises, and improve access to services. Central features of this project were its emphases upon establishing a culture of collaboration and sustaining the coalition by promoting commitment and local ownerships among the constituencies. Janicki (1996) and Janicki et al. (1996) in New York built a coalition of the New York State Office on Aging, the New York ARC, institutions of higher education, and a number of the state's Area Agencies on Aging to conduct outreach to older families caring for adults with developmental disabilities and to introduce individuals so identified to local aging and developmental services. In the Partners III Project in which the author was involved, Ansello (1996a, 1996b) and colleagues (Ansello et al., 1997) used a university-based center on aging in a "non-threatening, neutral brokering role" (Ansello & Eustis, 1992) between aging and developmental disabilities organizations. The project developed coalitions in Maryland and Virginia that would field test the implementation of a cumulative model for intersystem cooperation that was built from the successes of a half-dozen earlier collaborations, including one on independent living for older adults with visual impairments. The project identified three basic ingredients essential to meaningful cooperation across the systems:

1. Formal "top down" and "bottom up" mechanisms for collaboration must be in place statewide and locally.
2. Outreach strategies must be implemented that enable outreach to be a bridge to caregivers and consumers carrying traffic both ways, that is, information out to them and data back to agencies.
3. Activities must be conducted that build the capacities of formal providers of assistance (agency staffs), informal providers (family and friends), and older adults with developmental disabilities to identify and use appropriate resources that maximize the functioning of these older adults in the community.

LOCAL FOCUS

The thrust in both aging and disabilities is toward more and more local arenas of operation. The leadership and funding support for aging and developmental disabilities is not what it once was at the federal level. Even these previous levels of commitment were meager, but they are desirable compared to current circumstances. The Administration on Aging has had its discretionary grants program under Title IV of the Older Americans Act virtually eliminated by Congress, and with it went gerontology career preparation, field-initiated research, and model programs development. Overall appropriations for Title III services (senior centers, congregate meals, preventive health) have risen only modestly. Support for Geriatric Education Centers, funded through the Bureau of Health Professions, has been flat, which in itself is a victory of sorts. Creative funding streams for older people with developmental disabilities may be possible through the National Health Service Corps or the National Institute of Mental Health. These prospects, however, remain to be explored. Similarly, support for aging and vision rehabilitation has been episodic, at best, with little federal support for research on vision impairment in later life, for public education initiatives, or for independent living for post-working-age persons who are blind (see Chapter 8).

Overall, the focus of attention for support of aging and developmental disabilities initiatives seem to be shifting from the federal government to state governments, which are being handed both funded and unfunded mandates for services, training, and evaluation, along with requirements for the degree of efficiency to be achieved. Medicaid funding serves as an example, as it is a mix of federal and state monies. Rising Medicaid health expenditures have hastened the development by the states of state-managed care programs, as this joint program is rapidly consuming more and more of the states' budgets (Smith, Cotter, & Rossiter, 1996).

Within the state, this devolution of responsibility often continues. Local governments are being given more responsibility by the state for the administration of social, adult protective, mental health, and developmental disabilities services. The implications for the fields of aging and disabilities include an adjustment to a more local focus. Representatives from state and local government should sanction, indeed, participate in, collaborations between systems. This would create the "top down" and "bottom up" support required for coalitions to succeed in meeting their goals. At the same time, this localization of focus encourages small-scale initiatives that risk little financially while engaging important players who will remain a part of the solution after a period of funding has ended.

Experiences in the Partners Projects reinforce that while "top down" support is helpful in advancing cooperation among agencies, implementation of that cooperation in the form of purposeful activities is a local function. The Partners III Project's integrated model of service to older adults with developmental disabilities (Ansello et al., 1997) has as its most essential component the creation of an Area Planning and Service Committee (APSC) which covers a defined geographic area, usually a county in urbanized areas or a number of counties allied with an Area Agency on Aging. The APSC identifies local needs, sets local goals, and maximizes local resources. For example, in Virginia, local APSCs and the statewide Professional/Consumer Advocacy Council (PCAC) of the Partners III Project helped to conceptualize and pass legislation to benefit family caregivers of family members with two or more ADL impairments, by providing them with a $500 annual grant that could be used to purchase respite care, home-delivered meals, or anything else of the caregiver's choosing. The APSCs and PCAC secured patronage to introduce the bill in the Virginia General Assembly and obtained bipartisan sponsorship. The committee fomented grassroots support for the bill and testified on its behalf. The process of conceptualization, introduction of legislation, and advocacy reinforced the connections among the members of the partnership. Strategizing became a unifying experience for its diverse members.

PRINCIPLES OF COLLABORATION

Models of collaboration between aging and disabilities have been tested and may be applied. Exploration precedes linkages between and within the fields. In some communities, even across some states, the aging and disabilities fields are still largely unaware of the details about the other. When exploration does occur, it is seldom due to idle curiosity, but rather owes its existence to some perceived benefit from collaboration and to some person or persons who provided the spark.

The several model projects on intersystem collaboration referred to earlier have produced results from which lessons may be derived with respect to the efficacy of linkages. Again, the projects cited focused on lifelong, developmental disabilities and aging, but the principles that led to success seem appropriate and relevant to initiatives in vision rehabilitation and aging.

Linkages between the fields need to be purposeful. For example, collaboration may occur across or within fields in order to identify persons previously unknown who have particular characteristics, such as aging with mental retardation or dually diagnosed with certain conditions; or in order to conduct cross-training for staff, so that aging agency personnel can learn about particular developmental disabilities and vice versa; or in order to provide information and referral assistance to family caregivers of aging adults with lifelong disabilities.

Linkages should produce a new neutral entity, such as the area planning and service committee, one not belonging to or perceived to be "owned" by either or any of the fields being brought into collaboration. This does not necessarily mean the creation and administration of a new, funded bureaucracy, which would be far too impractical and politically unlikely. Rather, the units entering into a collaboration create in concept a new entity, such as the Area Planning and Service Committees mentioned earlier, that is born fresh and favors no parent, so cooperation can occur without fear of a hidden agenda. Printing the new entity's own stationery, even through desktop publishing, confirms the collaboration.

Commitment to the collaboration works better if put into writing, specifying who, what, and for how long an organization is obliging itself to the new enterprise. Having an inspired group leader, one zealous for broadened linkages, is a boon, for the collaboration's members are venturing into new territory.

The collaborators need to set activities that are achievable, so some success is manifest to the members in a reasonable time. In the context of a collaborative entity, the principle of setting successive approximations to a goal means that actions may be allocated among the members, with the accomplishment of each approximation reinforcing the whole.

Linkages are a process rather than an end to themselves. Membership and energy levels are fluid. The Partners III Project (Ansello et al., 1997) identified three basic ingredients for nurturing this process:

1. Some formal means of collaboration for on-going communication between the systems at both the state level, as in memoranda of agreement and statewide advocacy committees, and the local level, especially the creation of a neutral entity such as the Area Planning and Service Committee mentioned earlier.
2. Strategies for outreach to older adults with developmental disabilities and their informal caregivers who provide community-based assistance. Outreach might include resource fairs, home visitor surveys, focus groups, telephone surveys, and other initiatives.
3. Methods for building the capacities of formal providers of assistance (agency staffs), informal providers (families and friends), and older adults with developmental disabilities to identify and use appropriate resources that maximize the community functioning of these older adults. Capacity-building activities might include cross-training of staff, training in self-care and advocacy for consumers and informal caregivers, integration of elders with developmental disabilities into community services, and internships across systems for planners, policymakers, direct service providers, and managers. The cross-system internships prove especially valuable for learning how the "other" system works.

Linkages fare better when their focus is local. As helpful as commitment is at the state level, the ultimate beneficiaries of collaboration—namely, consumers and caregivers—live in neighborhoods. Keeping the composition of the neutral entity or Area Planning and Service Committee essentially local means that numbers do not become unwieldy, and the committee's successes become readily apparent in the community, thereby priming greater commitment from the partnering organizations.

Linkages tend to produce an economy that reduces the level of funding required to produce successes from collaboration. Monetary requirements for the collaboration are often greatly overestimated. In evaluating the five field tests of its integrated model in Maryland and Virginia, the Partners III Project learned that participants considered only a modest amount of money, $5,000 a year or less in total, necessary to implement this intersystem collaboration (Ansello et al., 1997). Much more critical, participants said, was for agencies to commit personnel to the process over time. With several partnering organizations in collaboration, the monetary requisite becomes shared and affordable, but, more importantly, the collaboration obviates many expenses through its reciprocity (e.g., staff cross-training is often accomplished without cost because of diverse expertise within the membership of the APSC; also, add-on mailings reduce or eliminate costs of outreach).

CONCLUSION

The evolutions of the aging of the nation and the longevity of persons with serious disabilities have not only produced a situation in which individuals grow old with disabilities but have also drawn attendant fields or systems into contact with each other. In some places, this contact is an intersection. Entering it unalert can be dangerous. Fortunately, those at the intersection of vision rehabilitation and aging can benefit from experiences of other travelers. A number of model projects and demonstrations have explored this intersection and have mapped ways of negotiating it. Their work suggests that collaboration in practice and in policy development can produce appreciable benefits for older adults with disabilities, family caregivers, and the respective systems. Policy implications are robust. Not the least of these is that collaborations across and within systems can produce more effective resource management, while serving consumers more effectively. These results are especially salient for policymakers, as the devolution of responsibilities related to aging and disabilities places more burdens upon state and local governments. Policymakers can be reassured in the relatively modest financial commitments required to instigate these collaborations but must reconcile themselves to the rather novel potential accoutrements of the collaborative process, including having agencies sharing some decision-making and endorsing another agency or organization in its work, when this other unit may be a competitor for governmental appropriations and public awareness.

The obstacles to collaborative practice and policy development are substantial. A "crisis du jour" mentality freezes many human service systems in their current mode of responding. Networks of planners, service providers, and advocates for persons who have been marginalized by others may see themselves as marginalized; and so they strive to hold on to what little they have and avoid initiatives they fear may jeopardize it. Family caregiving and self-care challenge the prevailing concept of chronic or long-term care. Collaborations may represent a risk, because they represent a change from the norm for members of the systems. Entering into cooperative ventures across and within systems calls for insight and creativity, as well as risk-taking. The demographic imperative of longer life expectancies, including those with lifelong and late-onset disabilities, and the increasing demands being placed upon public resources would seem to urge thoughtful examination of the intersection of aging and disabilities.

REFERENCES

American Association of Retired Persons & The Travelers Foundation. (1988). *A national survey of caregivers: Final report*. Washington, DC: Authors.

Anonymous. (1998). The economic and budget outlook: Fiscal years 1999–2008. *Medical Benefits, 15*(5), 1–2.

Ansello, E. F. (1996a). Partners III: Testing a model for aging and disabilities intersystem cooperation. Twenty-Second Annual Meeting of the Association for Gerontology in Higher Education.

Ansello, E. F. (1996b). Partners III: Real-world testing of a model for intersystem cooperation. 120th Annual Meeting of the American Association on Mental Retardation.

Ansello, E. F., Coogle, C. L., & Wood, J. B. (1997). *Partners: Building intersystem cooperation in aging with developmental disabilities*. Richmond, VA: Virginia Center on Aging.

Ansello, E. F., & Eustis, N. N. (Eds.) 1992. *Aging and disabilities: Seeking common ground*. Amityville, NY: Baywood.

Ansello, E. F., & Rose, T. (1989). *Aging and lifelong disabilities: Partnership for the twenty-first century*. Palm Springs, CA: Elvirita Lewis Foundation.

Ansello, E. F., Wells, A. I., & Zink, M. J. (1989). The Partners Project: Research and training on aging and developmental disabilities. Forty-second Annual Scientific Meeting of the Gerontological Society of America.

Callahan, D. (1987). *Setting limits: Medical goals in an aging society.* New York: Simon & Schuster.

Clark, P. G., & Susa, C. B. (in press). Promoting personal, familial, and organizational change through futures planning: Theory and practice. In M. P. Janicki & E. F. Ansello (Eds.), *Community supports for aging adults with lifelong disabilities.* Baltimore: Brookes.

Coogle, C. L., Ansello, E. F., Wood, J. B., & Cotter, J. J. (1995). Partners II—serving older persons with developmental disabilities: Obstacles and inducements to collaboration among agencies. *Journal of Applied Gerontology, 14*(3), 275–288.

Coogle, C. L., Ansello, E. F., Wood, J. B., & Cotter, J. J. (1997). *"Hot button" issues for 1997: State agencies serving older adults with DD tell us their concerns.* Eighteenth Annual Meeting of the Southern Gerontological Society.

Coppola, K. M., Danks, J. H., Ditto, P. H., & Smucker, W. D. (1998). Perceived benefits and burdens of life-sustaining treatments: Differences among elderly adults, physicians, and young adults. *Journal of Ethics, Law, and Aging, 4*(1), 3–13.

Cotter, J. J., Ansello, E. F., & Wood, J. B. (1992). Final report: Improving services to older persons with developmental disabilities: Policy, training, services. Richmond, VA: Virginia Department for the Aging.

Doty, P., Jackson, M. E., & Crown, W. (1998). The impact of female caregivers' employment status on patterns of formal and informal eldercare. *The Gerontologist, 38*(3), 331–341.

Factor, A. R. (1996). *Building coalitions to bridge the aging and developmental disabilities networks.* Forty-ninth Annual Scientific Meeting of the Gerontological Society of America.

Gilson, S. F., & Netting, F. E. (1997). When people with pre-existing disabilities age in place: Implications for social work practice. *Health & Social Work, 22*(4), 290–298.

Goldhagen, D. (1996). *Hitler's willing executioners.* New York: Knopf.

Janicki, M. P. (1996). *Area Agencies on Aging as the means for outreach and services to older caregivers.* Forty-ninth Annual Scientific Meeting of the Gerontological Society of America.

Janicki, M. P., Bishop, K. M., Cannon, N., Davidson, P., Force, L., Grant-Griffith, L., Le Pore, P., Lucchino, R., McCallion, P., & Schwartz, A. (1996). *Area Agencies on Aging as the means for outreach and services to older caregivers.* 120th Annual Meeting of the American Association on Mental Retardation.

Mittelman, M. S., Ferris, S. H., Schulman, E., Steinberg, G., & Levin, B. (1996). A family intervention to delay nursing home placement of patients with

Alzheimer's disease. *Journal of the American Medical Association, 276*(21), 1725–1731.

National Alliance for Caregiving and American Association of Retired Persons. (1997). *Family caregiving in the U.S.: Findings from a national survey.* Washington, DC: Authors.

Pernick, M. (1996). *The black stork: Eugenics and the death of "defective" babies in American medicine and motion pictures since 1915.* New York: Oxford University Press.

Smith, W. R., Cotter, J. J., & Rossiter, L. F. (1996). System change: Quality assessment and improvement for medical managed care. *Health Care Financing Review, 17*(4), 97–115.

Sterns, E., Heller, T., Sterns, H. L., Factor, A., & Miklos, S. (1994). *Person-centered planning for later life: A curriculum for adults with mental retardation.* Akron, OH: RRTC on Aging with Mental Retardation, The University of Illinois at Chicago and The University of Akron.

Sterns, H. L., Kennedy-Hart, E. A., Sed, C. M., & Heller, T. (In press). Later life planning and retirement. In M. P. Janicki & E. F. Ansello (Eds.), *Community supports for aging adults with lifelong disabilities.* Baltimore: Brookes.

Strommel, M., Collins, C. E., & Given, B. A. (1994). The costs of family contributions to the care of persons with dementia. *The Gerontologist, 34*(2), 199–205.

U.S. General Accounting Office. (1998). Long term care: baby boom generation presents financial challenges (No. T-HEHS-98–107). Washington DC: Author.

Zola, I. K. (1988). Aging and disability: Towards a unifying agenda. *Educational Gerontology, 14*(5), 365–388.

CHAPTER 9

Policy and Funding for Aging and Vision Rehabilitation Services

Lorraine Lidoff

Visual impairment is more prevalent than Alzheimer's disease (Crews, 1991; The Lighthouse, Inc., 1995; U.S. General Accounting Office, January 1998) and almost as feared as cancer (Horowitz, Reinhardt, Brennan, & Cantor, 1997), yet is largely unrecognized by the public. Although the term *legal blindness* is somewhat familiar, it is an arbitrary construct that really tells very little about how vision affects an individual's functioning (see Chapter 4).

Although much is known about dealing with the effects of vision loss, here, too, there are great gaps: treatable eye disease and correctable refractive error often go untreated (Horowitz, Balstreri, Stuen, & Fangmeier, 1993; Marx, Werner, Feldman, & Cohen-Mansfield, 1994; Tielsch, in press). The established techniques of vision rehabilitation are virtually unknown to the public, to the service providers who work with older adults—the majority of the visually impaired population, to health care providers, and often even to eye care physicians (The Lighthouse, Inc., 1995).

Visual impairment is a physical problem with enormous consequences for an individual's mobility, communication skills, social and vocational life, and ability to carry out ordinary activities of daily living—on a level with the consequences of a stroke or a broken hip. Yet there is no significant, stable funding stream for older people's vision rehabilitation, comparable to that which exists through Medicare and private health insurance for restorative therapies for a broken hip or a stroke (Lidoff, 1997).

Something is very wrong with this picture. The first question is Why? and the second is What needs to be done about it?

The answer to Why? emerges from a look at various systems and groups that might be expected to "own" the problem but thus far have not done so. One of these systems, health care, is presented as a case in point, with a detailed examination of the reasons that vision rehabilitation has not historically been included, as well as recent efforts to change the situation. The closing section of this chapter responds to the question of what needs to be done, outlining a substantial public policy agenda for the survival of vision rehabilitation.

WHOSE PROBLEM IS THIS, ANYWAY?

Older persons who are visually impaired do not fit neatly into any existing service system. The aging network—literally tens of thousands of providers of services and advocacy across the country—tends to think in terms of generic social services, rather than disease-specific or condition-specific services. (Alzheimer's disease is the exception, as is discussed later in this chapter.) Such generic services, for example, meals, transportation, and care management, might be quite appropriate for an older individual with vision impairment. However, these services often fail to reach those who are physically and emotionally isolated by their condition and to accommodate to their special communication, mobility, and safety needs. And State Units on Aging and Area Agencies on Aging are often unaware of the specialized vision rehabilitation services that exist in their own planning and service areas (Stuen, 1991).

The federal–state rehabilitation system focuses the great majority of its resources on "working age" adults and employment outcomes, that is, rehabilitating the individual to be able to work and actually placing him or her in a job. State rehabilitation agencies can pay for "homemaker closures," that is, closing an individual client's case by rehabilitating that person to live independently at home. Some state agencies have used this flexibility to serve older people who were legally blind. However, federal law and state policies are now reducing homemaker closures and focusing vocational rehabilitation dollars much more strictly on employment outcomes. Dedicated funding for independent living services for older individuals who are blind within the rehabilitation system under Title VII, Chapter 2 of the Rehabilitation Act of 1973, as amended is minuscule in relation to the need. For fiscal year 1998, the federal appropriation was a total of $10.9 million for all states and territories, and it was increased to $15 million for fiscal year 2000.

The nationwide network of independent living centers, which do see independent living as their primary goal, is not disability specific. In fact, independent living center staff are often not expert in vision loss as a disabling condition and in the specific skills that a visually impaired person must acquire in order to regain independence. The wheelchair symbol, which has become the accepted emblem of accessibility for persons with disabilities, perhaps inadvertently expresses a particular frame of reference. And most independent living centers focus on consumer empowerment rather than direct provision of services. Self-direction and autonomy are concepts that cannot be fully realized for people who are blind or visually impaired without adequate sources of necessary skills training and assistive devices to enable them to achieve independence.

The health care system, as already noted, pays for occupational and physical therapy for other physical conditions. It would appear to be the natural payer for rehabilitative services for older—or at least non-employment-bound—adults who lose their vision. However, only very recently have there begun to be any breakthroughs at all in persuading health system payers to cover vision rehabilitation.

WHERE IS THE CONSUMER VOICE?

Since the aging, rehabilitation, and health care systems are not addressing vision rehabilitation, why are consumers themselves not demanding services? The majority of individuals with severe vision impairment are older people, often very old people with multiple health problems. Vision loss affects every area of one's life; it can be devastating and very isolating. Is it reasonable to expect such a vulnerable group to organize and speak for itself? The case of Alzheimer's disease may provide an instructive parallel. It was not the individuals with dementia who converted the name of an obscure German physician into a household word. It was Dr. Robert Butler, the charismatic first director of the National Institute on Aging, who made Alzheimer's disease a research priority and encouraged the development of advocacy on a national scale. Services began to be created for people with Alzheimer's disease, as well as for family members whose lives also were profoundly affected by the disease. The private sector Alzheimer's Association now has a powerful voice, and there are local associations and caregiver support groups in communities across the country. Celebrity spokespersons have added glitz and clout.

To date, no such high-profile champion has emerged for older adults with vision impairment. The large consumer organizations in the "blindness" field, which have had considerable legislative influence, have focused on the working-age population and have not taken up the cause of older people. (Even visually impaired children have only relatively recently gained a national advocate—the National Association of Parents of the Visually Impaired.) Is there unintended ageism here? An implicit preference for employment over other forms of productivity? Pessimism about older people's ability to learn? Devaluation of the relatively small gains that an older person may make via rehabilitation—small gains that can make a very significant difference in that individual's life (Williams, 1984)?

One encouraging development is the growth of consumer support groups. For example, since Lighthouse International (formerly The Lighthouse Inc.) began to survey such groups in 1989 and serve as a national clearinghouse for these groups, their numbers have increased from 425 to nearly 850 across the country (personal communication from the Lighthouse International Information and Resource Service, 4/15/98). The groups focus on self-help, mutual support, and information exchange. They have the potential to be a network for advocacy, too, and some support groups have already been active in promoting legislation that would expand vision rehabilitation services and funding.

Two national organizations have taken up the challenge. Lighthouse International has been a source of valuable research, education, and consumer information through its National Center on Vision and Aging and its Arlene R. Gordon Research Institute. Some members of the Lighthouse-led National Vision Rehabilitation Cooperative, which was established by private agencies around the country that wanted to improve services and funding for older adults with vision impairment, are now pioneering a national managed care provider network. The American Foundation for the Blind (AFB) also has provided educational materials and rallied the field through its annual Josephine L. Taylor Leadership Institute. Both Lighthouse International and AFB have tackled the problem of lack of knowledge through national public awareness campaigns to bring vision loss and vision rehabilitation to the public's attention. But this is only a beginning.

PUBLIC POLICY TRENDS

Stepping beyond the vision rehabilitation field to the broader public policy arena, several major trends affect the potential for vision rehabilitation to gain financial support in the near future. The first of these is cost-cutting fervor. In an effort to trim government spending and balance the federal budget, funding for human services was first cut deeply and now is being held nearly level. Funding for health care has been tightened, too, and is now growing at a much-decreased rate. Despite the much-discussed "demographic imperative" and "graying of America," this is a bad time to be seeking more money to address the need for vision rehabilitation services.

Advocates for vision rehabilitation have been unsure what tack to take in this environment. Should high prevalence numbers be used to show that this is a major issue that demands attention? For example, the *Lighthouse National Survey on Vision Loss* (1995) found that 13.5 million adults age 45 and over report moderate or severe vision impairment. Or should much lower numbers, derived in other ways, be used to argue that this is a relatively small problem that will not cost society too much to address? For example, Nelson and Dimitrova (1993) estimated that only 4.3 million Americans of any age were severely visually impaired in 1990. In any case, the numbers will become much larger as the population ages, and the potential price tag will rise, too.

The second trend is privatization. The private sector is taking over responsibilities that formerly were handled by the government, making meeting human needs subject to the profit motive and market forces. The philosophical change is particularly visible in health care: managed care organizations have described their business as managing health care *costs,* rather than managing health *care* (though a more humanistic note is beginning to arise in the face of intense competition to sign up and retain customers). Vision rehabilitation agencies, other than those whose endowments make them financially independent, must change the way they think and become more business-oriented in their operations if they hope to survive.

The third trend is accountability. Payers are demanding results. Working hard and complying with process requirements are no longer enough; providers must produce and document specified outcomes. The basic outcome that funders want from vision rehabilitation services, reasonably enough, is functional improvement for the individual. But some funders, especially in the health care system, also are expecting rehabilitation services to result in cost savings through reduced use of more expensive services, for example, hospital days.

The fourth trend is consumer empowerment. Consumers are asserting their own expectations for and control over services. Characteristic of the demanding "baby boom" generation, and exemplified by the independent living movement, consumer empowerment is becoming a force in health and human services. It serves as a counterweight to the cost-cutting and privatization trends, insisting on quality as well as efficiency. Here consumers and nonprofit providers, with their tradition of caring and quality, have common ground. Consumer empowerment interacts, too, with the accountability trend by promoting outcomes that are defined and valued by the consumer, not just the payer. Again, consumers and providers will be most effective if they work closely together in communicating with payers.

HEALTH SYSTEM PAYMENT FOR VISION REHABILITATION

Though the health care system has not historically been a major payer for vision rehabilitation services, it is a logical source of funding, especially for the growing population of visually impaired older adults. Vision loss is a physical health problem, as already stated, and it has a pervasive impact on an individual's ability to function, comparable to the impact of a stroke or a serious injury.

Some reimbursement has been available for clinical low vision services provided by an ophthalmologist or an optometrist. In some states, the Medicaid program will pay for some low vision devices. Psychological services needed to help an individual make the difficult adjustment to vision loss are sometimes covered as clinical social work—although few mental health professionals are expert in the particular impacts of disability in a person's life. But even in this patchy picture, reimbursement levels have been unrealistically low, availability of services under Medicaid varies a great deal from state to state, and even Medicare coverage varies considerably from one carrier to another. Crucial therapeutic training to restore an individual's mobility and daily living skills has rarely been covered at all.

Part of the reason that vision rehabilitation has not been part of the health care system goes back to the beginning of modern rehabilitation services for people who lose their vision. Services and techniques evolved from programs for blinded veterans returning from World War II. Most of these relatively young men had few medical problems other than vision loss, and the specialized rehabilitation services developed for them were not considered part of broader medical rehabilitation (Wainapel, in press).

Part of the reason is based in the traditions of the "blind rehabilitation" field, which has seen its services as educational rather than therapeutic. Vision rehabilitation providers have been reluctant to adopt "the medical model," which they have seen as making them subject to physician oversight and restricting their independent judgment and practice. The national consumer organizations in the field have shared this aversion to the medical model, stating that blindness is not an illness and people who are blind are not patients, again with the implication of loss of autonomy.

Even for those vision rehabilitation providers who have sought reimbursement by Medicare and other health insurers, their practice (with the exception of clinical low vision services provided by eye care physicians) has generally lacked the rigor required by the health care system. Although the practice of orientation and mobility has historically been somewhat more rigorous than that of rehabilitation teaching, in reality the vision rehabilitation field has had nothing comparable to Medicare's standard of documentation for medical rehabilitation, linking precise diagnosis to quantified types and amounts of services to specified outcomes.

Further, credentialing of mobility instructors and rehabilitation teachers has been weak, compared to credentialing in the health care system. These professions are not licensed in any state (though a licensure effort is now advancing in New York). Certification has been self-administered by the field's professional organization, the Association for Education and Rehabilitation of the Blind and Visually Impaired (AER) and has not been based on a validated national examination (except for the new low vision therapist certification). Perhaps most significant, AER credentialing has not been recognized by any health care system entity.

A final reason that vision rehabilitation has not been covered by health system payers is that physicians, even most eye care physicians, are not aware of these services and do not refer patients for them. Vision rehabilitation providers frequently hear from their clients that an eye doctor has sent them off, saying, "There's nothing more I can do for you." Thus, the usual gateway to health care services has not opened onto vision rehabilitation.

During the period of ferment and debate opened up by President Clinton's proposal of a comprehensive health care reform plan in 1993, there seemed to be an opportunity for vision rehabilitation services to be included in the benefit package alongside parallel rehabilitation services. Advocates did succeed in getting "vision-related rehabilitation services" explicitly mentioned in one of the Congressional health care reform bills. However, this progress was erased when the entire health care reform effort unraveled, and the climate ended for extensive reform at the national level.

Nevertheless, various attempts to get Medicare, Medicaid, and private health insurers to pay for vision rehabilitation continued, first on a piecemeal basis and then via more comprehensive models. As noted previously, some reimbursement could be obtained by optometrists and ophthalmologists for part of the low vision examination. In a few states, Medicaid paid for vision rehabilitation as adult day health care; and in Rhode Island, Medicaid began to pay for a broader spectrum of vision rehabilitation services under its home and community-based services program. Reimbursement was occasionally obtained from private insurers by vision rehabilitation agencies for mobility instruction and rehabilitation teaching—usually on a case-by-case basis—by obtaining a physician's order and persuading the payer that the services were equivalent to occupational therapy. Some vision rehabilitation agencies have actually employed occupational therapists to provide vision rehabilitation services, and billed the services as occupational therapy.

Reimbursement for low vision devices has not been covered, except by some states' Medicaid programs. That route has been difficult, however, with complex procedures, long waiting times, and low levels of payment. The closed-circuit television (CCTV), which can be used to magnify and otherwise manipulate text to make it more readable for people with certain eye conditions (for example, macular degeneration), is an especially expensive item whose cost puts it out of reach of many potential users. Yet there are now a few examples of Medicare beneficiaries obtaining reimbursement on appeal for a CCTV as either a prosthetic device or durable medical equipment or both; and there was recently a successful appeal for coverage of a CCTV by Vermont's Medicaid program. (Lighthouse International is operating a clearinghouse to collect examples of coverage for CCTVs and promote more successes.)

Currently, three more comprehensive approaches have been developed to obtain health system payment for vision rehabilitation: the Hopkins model, the Comprehensive Outpatient Rehabilitation Facility (CORF), and the emerging managed care model.

The Hopkins Model

The Hopkins model is built on the work of Dr. Donald Fletcher, an ophthalmologist. Dr. Fletcher succeeded in persuading the U.S. Health Care Financing Administration that low vision was a condition that could potentially benefit from rehabilitation. He also convinced his own Medicare carrier to reimburse for rehabilitation teaching and mobility instruction, provided by staff in his employ and billed as "incident to" the physician's services. Dr. Fletcher used occupational therapists to provide rehabilitation teaching and orientation and mobility (O&M) instructors for mobility. The Lions Vision Research and Rehabilitation Center at Johns Hopkins has carried this approach still further, using AER-certified rehabilitation teachers and mobility instructors as an integral part of their low vision rehabilitation team, which is led by optometrists. They have carefully developed procedures and documentation to meet Medicare standards. (Two full issues, December 1995 and September 1996, of the *Journal of Vision Rehabilitation* were devoted to detailing this approach; see Massof et al., 1995, 1996.)

Through persistent advocacy and education, Johns Hopkins gained the support of their Medicare carrier's medical director, and initial denials of claims have since been reversed. The medical director of this carrier led a group of his colleagues who had been appointed by the Health Care Financing Administration to make recommendations regarding rehabilitation service codes. The group eventually issued a draft Local Coverage Policy guideline on low vision rehabilitation, which incorporates the concepts and codes of the Hopkins model. Each Medicare carrier across the country has the option to adopt such a guideline, adopt parts of it, or ignore it. Thus far, carriers in more than a dozen states have adopted it formally or informally—meaning that they will pay claims for services following this model. There is no requirement to use rehabilitation teachers and orientation and mobil-

ity instructors in the model: physicians may use occupational therapists if they choose, and reimbursement is higher for services billed as
occupational therapy than for services billed as "incident to" the physician's services. Also, "incident to" providers must work under a
physician's direct supervision, and thus, for example, rehabilitation
teaching services in a patient's home or mobility service on the street
would not be covered. It should be noted that this is a fee-for-service
model, although its conceptualization of vision rehabilitation as a
health care service should also be applicable in a capitated managed
care environment.

The CORF Model

The Comprehensive Outpatient Rehabilitation Facility is an entity
defined in the Medicare law as a distinct facility to offer a range of
medically necessary rehabilitation services in an outpatient setting. A
wide array of services may be furnished under a plan of treatment
established by a CORF physician. Covered services include physician
services, nursing, social and psychological services, physical therapy,
occupational therapy, respiratory therapy, speech and language
pathology, prosthetic and orthotic devices, durable medical equipment, drugs, supplies, and equipment. Note that for CORFs, the physician who defines and oversees the treatment plan must be an MD or
a DO, not an optometrist. Optometry services can be covered,
however.

The best known example of a CORF providing vision rehabilitation
services is the Jewish Guild for the Blind in New York. The Guild uses
physical therapists to provide mobility services and occupational
therapists to teach activities of daily living (Morse, in press). Although
the Guild does not do so, it may be possible to include the services of
mobility instructors and rehabilitation teachers as physician or occupational therapist extenders, similar to the "incident to" approach
already described. Reimbursement would be at the discretion of the
Medicare carrier. Because CORFs are required to offer a full range of
rehabilitation services, a critical element of financial success is maintaining a patient flow adequate to justify the specialized staff needed
to handle vision rehabilitation.

The Managed Care Model

As managed care has been rapidly taking over the health care system, it is clearly essential to develop models of vision rehabilitation that would be attractive to managed care organizations. Managed care organizations demand a high degree of efficiency and measurable outcomes—not only the achievement of rehabilitation goals, but also cost savings in other areas of health care utilization, especially hospital lengths of stay. For vision rehabilitation agencies, this requires extensive revamping of service delivery structures, financial management, and information systems.

The managed care model development effort that is farthest along to date is that of Lighthouse International. A package of services, procedures, and documentation is being developed to market to managed care organizations.

A number of member agencies of the National Vision Rehabilitation Cooperative have decided to join with Lighthouse International to establish the Lighthouse National Vision Rehabilitation Network. Through the high-quality reputations of participating agencies and the geographic coverage they offer, this provider network should have more marketing leverage with managed care organizations than any single agency could have on its own. Such a national effort holds the promise of setting the standard for vision rehabilitation service—not in the sense of a legislated national standard, as managed care is a market phenomenon (not a government program, like Medicare or Medicaid), but in the sense of a recognized emblem of quality.

The National Vision Rehabilitation Cooperative is now spearheading a legislative effort to make orientation and mobility specialists and rehabilitation teachers eligible providers under Medicare. If such legislation is enacted, it would complement and enhance any of the existing models.

A PUBLIC POLICY AGENDA

For vision rehabilitation to survive and thrive, given the problems outlined and in the context of broader policy trends, a substantial agenda must be carried out. One component of the agenda is that vision rehabilitation agencies themselves must adapt and change, as the discussion regarding the potential for health system coverage for services illustrates. To state it more generally, vision rehabilitation providers must learn to describe, structure, and document services in ways that are recognizable by the system from which they expect to be paid. If vision rehabilitation agencies succeed in adapting in this manner, the potential exists for provision of services to become an income stream rather than an expense—that is, agencies could operate as service-providing businesses instead of service-providing charities.

A second essential component of a public policy agenda is that the visibility of vision loss in the aging population, and of the vision rehabilitation services necessary to help restore independence, must be increased. Public education is necessary to generate informed demand for services. The education of physicians—ophthalmologists and optometrists, geriatricians, and primary care physicians—is absolutely necessary to generate adequate assessment of the individual's condition; treatment of conditions that are subject to remediation by surgery, medications, or prescription lenses; and referral to appropriate rehabilitation services.

Third, Area Agencies on Aging (AAAs), which have a broad advocacy responsibility to the entire older population, must become more responsive to the issue of vision impairment as it is clearly widespread among this age group. AAAs need to collect data on vision impairment and consequent needs as part of the mandated periodic needs assessment of their planning and service areas. Aging network outreach efforts should accommodate the special communication and mobility problems of visually impaired older people, as they accommodate the problems associated with other age-related disabilities. Care management and direct service staff should be trained to recognize signs of vision loss, to communicate effectively with people with vision impairment, and to make appropriate referrals.

Fourth, the real numbers of older people whose daily functioning is impaired by their vision loss must be ascertained, and those numbers used consistently in advocating for increased availability of services.

Fifth, outcomes must be defined for vision rehabilitation that are significant for consumers and credible to payers. In the health care system example, we see that services will be paid for only if they are demonstrably effective in restoring independent functioning and quality of life and help avert medical complications and injuries and hence costly hospital stays and other health care expenses. Thus the price of addressing the problem must be shown to be offset by the price of neglecting it.

Sixth, the consumer voice must be organized and educated. Existing support groups are a grassroots base for such advocacy. The families of older people who become visually impaired, and whose own lives are often greatly affected by their relatives' condition, are natural allies. An organization at the national level must take on the task of helping to raise the volume of the consumer voice.

This agenda requires a broad effort throughout the entire field to make vision rehabilitation visible to the health care system, potential consumers, and the public. The survival of vision rehabilitation in today's environment depends on bringing it into the mainstream of public policy.

*The author wishes to thank Cynthia Stuen, Lighthouse International Senior Vice President for Education and Training, and Karen Seidman, Lighthouse International Director of Continuing Education, for their valuable suggestions for this chapter.

REFERENCES

Crews, J. E. (1991). Measuring rehabilitation outcomes and the public policies on aging and blindness. In *Vision and aging: Issues in social work practice.* New York: Haworth, pp. 137–151.

Horowitz, A., Balistreri, E., Stuen, C., & Fangmeier, R. (1993). *Vision impairment among nursing home residents: Implications for physical and cognitive functioning.* Presented at the 46th Annual Scientific Meeting of the Gerontological Society of America, New Orleans, Louisiana.

Horowitz, A., Reinhardt, J. P., Brennan, M., & Cantor, M. (1997). *Aging and vision loss: Experiences, attitudes and knowledge of older Americans.* Final report to the Andrus Foundation. New York: The Lighthouse Inc.

Lidoff, L. (1997). Moving vision-related rehabilitation into the U.S. health care mainstream. *Journal of Visual Impairment & Blindness,* 90(2), 107–116.

The Lighthouse Inc. (1995). *The Lighthouse National Survey on Vision Loss: The experience, attitudes, and knowledge of middle-aged and older Americans.* New York: The Lighthouse Inc.

Marx, M. S., Werner, P., Feldman, R., & Cohen-Mansfield, J. (1994). The eye disorders of residents of nursing homes. *Journal of Visual Impairment & Blindness, 88*(5), 462–468.

Massof, R. W., Dagniele, G., Deremeik, J. T., DeRose, J. L., Alibhai, S. S., & Glasner, N. M. (1995). Low vision rehabilitation in the U.S. health care system. *The Journal of Vision Rehabilitation, 9,* 1–31.

Massof, R. W., Alibhai, S. S., Deremeik, J. T., Glasner, N. M., Baker, F., DeRose, J. L., & Dagniele, G. (1996). Low vision rehabilitation: Documentation of patient evaluation and management. *The Journal of Vision Rehabilitation, 10,* 1–31.

Morse, A. R. (in press). The Jewish Guild for the Blind: Comprehensive outpatient rehabilitation facility. In R. W. Massof & L. Lidoff, Eds. *Issues in low vision rehabilitation: Health care policy and service delivery.* New York: AFB Press.

Nelson, K. A. & Dimitrova, E. (1993). Severe visual impairment in the United States and in each state, 1990. *Journal of Visual Impairment & Blindness, 87,* 80–85.

Stuen, C. (1991). Awareness of resources for visually impaired older adults among the aging network. In *Vision and aging: Issues in social work practice.* New York: Haworth, pp. 165–175.

Tielsch, J. M. (in press). Prevalence of visual impairment and blindness in the United States. In R. W. Massof & L. Lidoff, , Eds. *Issues in low vision rehabilitation: Health care policy and service delivery.* New York: AFB Press.

United States General Accounting Office (January 1998). *Alzheimer's disease: Estimates of prevalence in the United States.* Publication number GAO-HEHS-98–16.

Wainapel, S. F. (in press). Low vision rehabilitation and rehabilitation medicine. In R. W. Massof & L. Lidoff, Eds. *Low vision rehabilitation: Health care policy and service delivery.* New York: AFB Press.

Williams, T. F. (1984). *Rehabilitation in the aging.* New York: Raven Press.

CHAPTER 10

Directions for Research in Aging and Vision Rehabilitation

Amy Horowitz and Cynthia Stuen

This chapter sets forth a research agenda relevant to psychosocial issues in aging, vision loss, and vision rehabilitation. As such, the discussion focuses on identifying what *is not* known about the experience of age-related vision loss and its rehabilitation rather than on what *is* known. In many respects, this represents a relatively easy task. Until very recently, the gerontological literature has ignored the specific implications of vision loss in later life, and the vision rehabilitation literature has ignored the elderly. In fact, although the elderly clearly represent the vast majority of persons with visual impairments (Kirchner, 1985; The Lighthouse Inc., 1995), the vision rehabilitation literature contains more than twice as many citations relating to children as it does to those relating to to older adults (Rosenbloom & Goodrich, 1997). Fortunately, in recent years there has been a change in this trend, with greater research attention being given to the specific issues, consequences, and interventions relevant to older adults who experience an age-related vision impairment. However, as is noted throughout this chapter, our empirical knowledge base continues to be characterized primarily by small-sample, cross-sectional studies, and therefore provides limited guidance regarding the long-term sequelae of vision loss in later life that can be generalized to the larger population of older people with visual impairments.

In the discussion that follows, we first address research needs relative to two broad but related questions that confront the field: (1) What are the processes and predictors of adaptation to an age-related vision impairment? and (2) What are the outcomes of vision rehabilitation interventions for older adults? Following this macro-level approach to identifying a research agenda in vision and aging, selected substantive topics are highlighted, along with relevant methodological issues. The chapter concludes with a brief discussion of the future outlook for research in aging, vision loss, and vision rehabilitation.

RESEARCH ON ADAPTATION TO AGE-RELATED VISION LOSS

A growing body of evidence underscores the profound consequences of a vision impairment for the physical and emotional well-being of older persons. This evidence is largely based on the gerontological literature, drawing from community samples and comparing elders who are visually impaired with their nonimpaired counterparts. Vision impairment has been found associated with greater functional disability in activities of daily living (ADLs), lower levels of social activity, and reduced mobility (see, e.g., Branch, Horowitz, & Carr, 1989; Carabellese et al., 1993; Golden, Teresi, & Gurland, 1984; Havlik, 1986; Heinemann, Colorez, Frank, & Taylor, 1988; Salive et al., 1994). In fact, vision impairment appears to have a more severe impact on everyday functioning compared to other physical impairments (Ford et al., 1988; Furner, Rudberg, & Cassel, 1995; Verbrugge & Patrick, 1995) and also has been found to increase the risk for decline in functional ability over time, even after other risk factors such as age, gender, cognitive status, and baseline functioning are controlled (LaForge, Spector, & Sternberg, 1992; Mor et al., 1989; Salive et al., 1994). Data from population-based studies of elders living in the community also indicate that visually impaired elders are at increased risk of poorer psychological well-being and affective disorders, especially depression, than their nonimpaired peers (Branch et al., 1989;

Carabellese et al., 1993; Golden et al., 1984; Lee, Gomez-Marin, & Lam, 1996).

These functional and psychological consequences of a vision loss in later life are not inevitable or invariable for any given older person, however. Clinical experience has indicated that psychosocial adaptation to age-related vision loss exists along a continuum, ranging from acceptance and functional compensation to denial, dependence, and despondence. Adaptation also needs to be conceptualized as a dynamic process that undergoes change over time in response to changes in the biopsychosocial environment of the individual, rather than as an end point in adjustment.

Although this view of adaptation to a vision loss in later life is consistent with current practice wisdom in the rehabilitation service system, only a paucity of empirical data are available to document how older people who are visually impaired are distributed on this continuum at different stages in their experience of vision loss or the factors that are associated with more or less successful adaptation. This dearth of information is a function of both the relatively few research studies that address adaptation to age-related vision loss and the conceptual and methodological limitations of much of the existing research in this field. Such limitations include:

- ◆ The atheoretical approach that has characterized many of the empirical investigations in the field
- ◆ The challenges and controversies in developing conceptual and operational definitions of "adaptation" relevant to older adults
- ◆ Reliance on relatively small, select samples drawn from service utilizing populations, which limits both the generalizability of findings and the statistical power of multivariate analyses needed to identify significant unique predictors of adaptation
- ◆ Primary reliance on cross-sectional designs that can offer only a "slice in time" in the adaptation process.

Each of these issues is discussed in turn.

Model of Adaptation

Although there are many theoretical models applicable to the study of adaptation to age-related vision loss, a useful conceptual framework is the stress and coping model of Lazarus and Folkman (1984). This model has been widely used in the extensive body of gerontological research addressing the impact of various chronic physical impairments on psychological well-being in old age. In simplified form, the stress and coping model (see Figure 1) posits that when an individual is confronted with a stressor (e.g., vision impairment), his or her personal resources (e.g., coping strategies and appraisals), in addition to social resources (e.g., informal and formal support), are crucial in influencing adaptation outcomes (e.g., adaptation, psychosocial well-being) (Lazarus & DeLongis, 1983; Lazarus & Folkman, 1984). In addition, (although not explicitly reflected in Figure 1), the individual brings to the situation a range of predisposing factors (e.g., sociodemographic characteristics, general health status) that interact with both the stressor and the personal and social resources to further influence adaptation.

Although this model represents a useful conceptual framework to ground research in adaptation to vision loss among the elderly, it is important not to underestimate its inherent complexity when applied in research designs. Using this model, the researcher has important

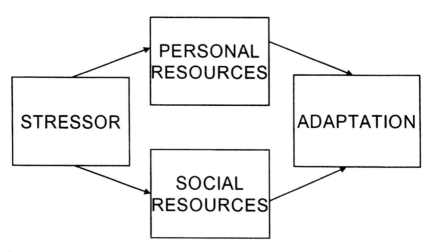

Figure 10.1
Model of Stress and Coping of Adaptation

Source: Adapted from Lazarus, R. S., & Folkman, S. (1984). *Stress, appraisal and coping.* New York: Springer.

conceptual and operational decisions to make. For example, the stressor of visual impairment can be defined by clinically measured severity (e.g. acuity, contrast sensitivity, etc.), subjectively assessed severity, type of eye disease(s), type of functional vision loss, and/or time since impairment onset. Personal resources may include measures of coping strategies used, subjective appraisals of the vision loss, perceptions of self-efficacy or personal mastery, locus of control, and/or a variety of personality traits. Social resources can be both informal and formal support components. Informal support may be measured by the availability of family, friends, and neighbors, the amount of contact with these support system members, the amount of assistance provided, and/or the quality of such relationships. Formal support may involve the use of general services available to the elderly in the community (e.g., homemakers, transportation services, senior centers) as well as the use of specific vision rehabilitation services. Obviously, no one study can include all possible measures pertaining to the different components of the model, and choices must be made by the individual researcher based on their particular research focus, as well as the prior research findings regarding potentially important predictors of adaptation.

Although we have recommended the stress and coping model as a useful conceptual framework to study adaptation to vision loss among the elderly, it is important to note that several investigators (e.g., Crews, 1991; Wahl & Oswald, in press) have argued for the expansion of this model to include environmental characteristics as well. This perspective recognizes that adaptation is not only "person centered," but is also a function of the physical or social environmental contexts in which the visual impairment is experienced and adaptation occurs. Thus, the extent to which the environment is "friendly" to the visually impaired older person, as well as the extent to which the individual is able to actively address and shape his or her relationship with the physical environment, represent important areas for both conceptual and empirical attention. Disability clearly represents an interaction between an individual with an impairment and the environment rather than solely a deficit of an individual (National Council on Disability, 1998). Thus, there is a need for both ". . . person-centered as well as the environment-centered view of visual impairment in order to fully understand visual impairment, its psychosocial consequences and the appropriate means of prevention and rehabilitation" (Wahl & Oswald, in press).

Measuring Adaptation

But the greatest challenge for the field of aging and vision impairment is the conceptualization and measurement of psychosocial adaptation. A major barrier to research in adaptation to vision impairment has been the lack of an appropriate, psychometrically tested measure of adaptation relevant to the elderly with vision loss in later life. Unfortunately, most of the previous research in adaptation to vision loss, including the instruments used to measure adaptation, have focused on young and middle-aged populations within the context of vocational rehabilitation (e.g., Dodds, Bailey, Pearson, & Yates, 1991; Dodds, Ferguson, Ng, Hawes, & Yates, 1994; Dodds, Flannigan, & Ng, 1993; Ehmer & Needham, 1979; Fitting, 1954; Lukoff & Whiteman, 1970; Needham & Ehmer, 1980). In lieu of a specific measure of adaptation to late-life vision loss, other researchers have relied, exclusively or in part, on global measures of well-being in later life. Drawing upon a long history of gerontological research, well-being in later life typically has been defined either globally, as the congruence between desired and achieved lifetime goals and measured through life satisfaction or morale scales, or in terms of one or more indicators of psychological status (e.g., depression, anxiety, self-esteem, etc.). In line with this tradition, Dodds et al. (1991) developed the Nottingham Adjustment Scale, a multidimensional measure drawn from selected items of existing scales and based on the conceptualization of adjustment to vision loss as being characterized by ". . . low levels of anxiety, an absence of depression, high self-esteem, a high sense of self-efficacy, a high sense of responsibility for recovery, a positive attitude towards visually impaired people and a high acceptance of one's visual disability" (p. 309). More recently, there have been efforts to develop domain-specific measures of adaptation to vision loss such as the Adaptation to Age-Related Vision Loss (AVL) scale (Horowitz & Reinhardt, 1998), the National Eye Institute's Visual Functioning Questionnaire (National Eye Institute, 1996) and the Functional Independence Measure for Blind Adults (Long, Crews, & Mancil, 1995). Each measure is in response to the identified need for standardized measures that specifically address vision-related, rather than global, well-being in later life that can be applied and compared across research studies. As Horowitz and Reinhardt (1998) argue, although adjustment to vision loss is a component of general well-being, it is not synonymous with adaptation to aging. Thus, domain-specific measures of adaptation to vision loss, when used in conjunction with more global measures of life satisfaction or psychological status, can provide a more complete picture of adaptation outcomes relative to the stressor of vision impairment in later life. These efforts to develop adaptation measures relevant to an older visually impaired population represent a welcome trend in the research literature. However, such research remains in its infancy and a long road still remains toward building a knowledge base in adaptation to age-related vision loss.

Broader Samples

Previous research in adaptation has also been limited by the nature of the samples studied. Most research has focused almost exclusively on populations utilizing rehabilitation services which is understandable given the ready availability of such persons for research recruitment. However, only a small percentage of older persons who could benefit from vision rehabilitation services are ever referred to or seek such services (The Lighthouse Inc., 1995). In ways still unknown (another fruitful area for future research), those who utilize rehabilitation services clearly differ from those who do not. It can also be safely assumed that the processes and outcomes of adaptation to the vision loss also differ for the latter group. How they differ remains an open question, however, given the dearth of research on individuals who do not utilize services. Kirchner (in press) has suggested that when samples are drawn from clients receiving services they tend to be biased toward those who are better off in terms of social supports and adaptation to the vision loss when compared to the entire visually impaired population, and therefore underestimate the consequences of vision impairment. Thus, it is important for future research to move out of the agency setting into the general community to identify and recruit samples to understand better the processes of adaptation for the broader population of older persons who are visually impaired.

Longitudinal Studies

Longitudinal studies in adaptation to vision loss in later life are also critically needed. As noted earlier, cross-sectional studies can provide only a "slice in time" view of the adaptation process. Yet, adaptation is a dynamic process, responding to changes in both the stressor (e.g., changes in level of visual impairment) and in the mediating personal and social resources available to the individual (e.g., changes in types of coping strategies over time) (Lazarus & DeLongis, 1983). In fact, an important related research need is to examine the relative change or stability in these personal and social factors and how they, in turn, influence changes in adaptation over time.

EVALUATION OF REHABILITATION OUTCOMES

From a policy and funding perspective, social and health-related services have clearly moved, even if somewhat reluctantly, into the "age of accountability." All such services are struggling with issues of standardized assessments, definition of appropriate outcomes, and measurement of short- and long-term effects of interventions. But the field of vision rehabilitation is making this move at an even slower pace than many other service fields. As Crews and Long (1997) note, the field of vision rehabilitation has little history or tradition in measuring rehabilitation outcomes. Kirchner (in press) suggests that the lag in the field of vision impairment may reflect the fact that its professionals have not been eligible for third-party reimbursement, as well as the constraints that many small vision rehabilitation agencies face in developing computerized information systems to facilitate data collection and analyses.

Whatever the past history has been in the evaluation of vision rehabilitation outcomes, rehabilitation professionals no longer have the luxury of saying they "do good" without the empirical data to support these claims. Ironically, one major impetus for the development of standardized outcomes measures and procedures comes from the managed care delivery and financing systems that are currently promulgating in the United States (Rosenbloom & Goodrich, 1997). Driven by goals of reducing costs in the most expensive modes of care (i.e, inpatient hospital and institutional long-term care), managed care programs are beginning to promote the less expensive, preventive health services, including rehabilitation services for the prevention of disability (Silverstone, 1998). Thus, one of the major challenges that researchers in vision impairment and rehabilitation currently face is the design of systematic evaluations of rehabilitation service interventions to provide empirical evidence of their value (Crews & Long, 1997; Horowitz & Reinhardt, in press; Kirchner, in press; Rosenbloom & Goodrich, 1997). But the key question then becomes, How does one define "value"?

Thus, defining relevant outcomes for vision rehabilitation has emerged as a priority for our research agenda. Outcome measures for rehabilitation services, including vision rehabilitation, need to be conceptualized as more than the mere acquisition of functional skills. Rather, measured outcomes need to be consistent with and reflect the broader goals of rehabilitation, including maximizing functional independence, fostering psychosocial adaptation to the disability, maintaining or regaining ability to fulfill age appropriate social roles, and enhancing overall quality of life.

Thus, outcomes must be conceptualized and measured on several levels. Clinical outcomes are the most basic level. In vision rehabilitation, these may include increased reading speed as a function of the use of a low vision device, successfully learning appropriate techniques of cane travel, and ability to use kitchen appliances. Successful clinical outcomes may or may not translate into successful outcomes on the second level of more global functional abilities, such as functional abilities in accomplishing basic personal care and instrumental activities of daily living (ADLs and IADLs). These more global activities would include, for example, ability to care for one's personal appearance, bathe and feed oneself, prepare meals, shop for groceries, travel within one's neighborhood, etc. Finally, outcomes must also address psychosocial adjustment and general quality of life. The measurement issues and options discussed in relationship to adaptation research are also relevant here and would include the need for measures of attitudes toward the vision impairment, global indicators of quality of life such as life satisfaction and morale, and affective states such as depressive and anxiety disorders. As Ringering and Amaral (in press) note, these goals, although conceptually distinct, can be expected to be interrelated in that ". . . success or failure in one category of outcomes effects the progress in reaching the other set of goals."

A word of caution is also in order in terms of outcome measurement. In this age of managed care and concerns about the rising costs of long-term care for the elderly, it is tempting to "oversell" the expected effects of vision rehabilitation relative to its effects on utilization of other health-related services. Although one may reasonably hypothesize that increased functional independence as a result of vision rehabilitation will lead to reduced need for home care service hours over the long run, claims of effects on prevention of hospital and nursing home care utilization are most probably overly optimistic, especially in the short term. Based on a vast body of research in gerontology, it is known that nursing home placement for elderly people is largely a function of the absence or "burn out" of family supports as well as specific conditions such as dementia and incontinence (see, e.g., Aneshensel, Pearlin, Mullan, Zarit, & Whitlatch, 1995; Freedman, Berkman, Rapp, & Ostfeld, 1994; Hanley, Alecxih, Wiener, & Kennell, 1990; Horowitz, 1985; McFall & Miller, 1992). Vision rehabilitation interventions are not necessarily targeted to those elders at most immediate risk of nursing home placement and therefore should not be expected to act to prevent or postpone nursing home care. To do so is to inevitably set the stage for failure.

Another issue relevant to measuring outcomes is the recognition that comorbidity is more the rule than the exception among older persons. Thus, functional disabilities that are exhibited may be a function of the vision impairment or may be related to another condition such as arthritis, or may result from the interaction of vision loss with other chronic conditions. Therefore, to isolate the effects of vision impairment on functional status it is important in the assessment and in the measurement of outcomes to clearly define which deficits are related to the vision impairment and thus can be affected by vision rehabilitation interventions. Research conducted at Lighthouse International (Horowitz, Leonard, & Reinhardt, 1996, 1997a,b; Horowitz, Reinhardt, McInerney, & Balistreri, 1984) found it very useful to use a follow-up question to each item assessing difficulty in a specific ADL and IADL task, inquiring "Is [the task] difficult primarily because of your vision problem, some other health problem, or a combination of vision and other health problems?" It was found that the vast majority of older persons are able to clearly identify the tasks in which their vision loss plays a role and those in which it does not. These data are important because only those functional areas that are affected by vision should be isolated for analyses of rehabilitation outcomes. For example, if problems with travel outside the home are a result of arthritis-related mobility restrictions, it would be unreasonable to expect that vision rehabilitation interventions will result in improvements in ability to travel independently. Although this is rather self-evident, it is often not explicitly reflected in current evaluation designs.

In addition to the importance of clearly defining and measuring rehabilitation outcomes on various levels, three other issues need to be considered in the evaluation of vision rehabilitation services. The first relates to the timing of post-service evaluations. Most current research studies have collected data at the conclusion of service provision. However, these data provide insight only into immediate post-service effects and are influenced by a "halo" effect surrounding the completion of the rehabilitation program. More important, both in terms of understanding service effectiveness and in policy relevance, is the retention of rehabilitation gains over time. This is an area in which almost no data are available. Ideally, follow-up takes place at 3- and 6-month post-service periods, as well as long-term follow-ups at 1 year or more. Thus, longitudinal designs are as important in evaluation studies as they are in studies of adaptation.

Second, in terms of evaluation designs, most existing research studies have depended on pretest/posttest designs. More rigorous experimental designs have seldom been used, largely because of difficulties in denying services to a nontreatment control group or difficulties in obtaining enough subjects who meet the eligibility criteria of a study (Crews & Long, 1997; Kirchner, in press). Experimental designs can in fact be fruitfully applied in the evaluation of vision rehabilitation services, however, primarily in terms of examining the relative effectiveness of different treatment protocols. Even as little systematic empirical data are available that document rehabilitation outcomes in general, many unanswered questions persist about the relative outcomes of different types of rehabilitation services and modes of delivering services. For example, experimental designs with random assignment to treatment groups could be used to examine the effectiveness of individual versus group methods of rehabilitation instrument, the added value of support groups for older adults in rehabilitation, as well as different instructional methods for the use of low vision aids. These types of studies are especially important as the field moves to a more critical examination of which services and techniques are most effective in producing desired outcomes and for varying groups of older persons.

Third, little attention has been given to the mechanisms underlying the effect of rehabilitation on psychosocial well-being among visually disabled elders. Given the well-documented relationship between functional disability and psychosocial well-being, a cogent argument, although still open to empirical investigation, can be made for hypothesizing that the primary pathway through which rehabilitation affects well-being is by improvements in levels of functional ability. Yet, the goal of rehabilitation is not only to maximize functional ability and stem functional decline, but also to facilitate adaptation to the disability and instill a sense of empowerment and control (Warren & Lampert, 1994). Thus, it can be hypothesized that the pathways by which rehabilitation interventions influence affective states also include the interventions' direct effects on attitudes toward the disability, feelings of self-efficacy and mastery, and use of coping strategies, as well as on social support relationships. These are hypotheses that require testing in order to advance our understanding of the processes of rehabilitation and their influence on quality of life outcomes.

PRIORITY AREAS FOR RESEARCH

In this section we turn to research needs in selected topics, all of which are relevant to the broader questions regarding adaptation to a vision loss in later life and rehabilitation outcomes. They are not intended to exhaust the range of substantive areas in which empirical data are sorely needed. Rather, they serve as examples of some of the more critical research issues and questions that we face in the field of aging and vision loss.

Family Support Systems

There is a rich research tradition in gerontology focusing on family caregiving to the frail and disabled elderly. Cumulative findings from three decades of gerontological research have consistently documented the importance of family members in providing emotional and instrumental support to older relatives, as well as the stresses experienced by the family as a consequence of caring for a disabled older relative (see, e.g., Aneshensel et al., 1995; Biegel & Blum, 1990; Biegel, Sales, & Schultz, 1991; Brody, 1985; Cantor & Little, 1985; George & Gwyther, 1986; Horowitz, 1985; Schulz, Visintainer, & Williamson, 1990; Stone, Cafferata, & Sangl, 1987). Much of this research, however, has focused on issues of family caregiving to elders with Alzheimer's disease or other cognitive disorders. The family support situations of the physically disabled but mentally intact elderly have received much less attention.

In particular, only a handful of research studies have examined the concerns and situations of families of elders with visual impairments (see, e.g., Crews & Frey, 1993; Dumas & Sadowsky, 1984; Goodman, Horowitz, Reinhardt, & Bird, 1996; Horowitz, Goodman, & Reinhardt, 1998). Findings from these studies point to the emotional stresses that families of visually impaired older adults experience, especially in regard to their concerns about the elder's safety and emotional well-being, and coming to terms with when, how, and how much to assist. Further empirical investigations into the concerns, reactions, and stresses experienced by families of elders with vision loss are critically needed, as such data would provide a foundation for the design of rehabilitation programs that incorporate a family-based model of rehabilitation practice. The latter is an important service priority, in light of increasing clinical evidence supporting the importance of family involvement, attitudes, and support during the rehabilitation process as well as in the retention of short-term and long-term rehabilitation gains (Becker & Kaufman, 1988; Dumas & Sadowsky, 1984; Kelly & Lambert, 1992; Moore, 1984; Osterweil, 1990; Silverstone, 1984; Youngblood & Hines, 1992).

However, both the gerontological and the vision rehabilitation research literature have virtually ignored the role families do, or may, play in the rehabilitation of their older relatives (Brody, 1986). Although research data are limited, existing evidence does provide support for the close relationship between the availability and quality of social supports and positive rehabilitation outcomes across a variety of health conditions such as stroke, hip fracture, arthritis, and heart disease (see, e.g., Cummings et al., 1988; Evans et al., 1987; Kaufman, Albright, & Wagner, 1987; Roberto, 1992; Thomas & Stevens, 1974). In studies specific to the elderly with vision impairments, similar trends regarding the importance of family supports in rehabilitation emerge. Horowitz & Reinhardt (1992) found that it was the quality of the relationship with a close family member that predicted the elder's adaptation to vision loss, rather than the mere availability of family members. A high level of family support has also been found associated with successful utilization of low vision optical devices (Greig, West, & Overbury, 1986) and better readjustment following a therapeutic group program (Emerson, 1981). Oppegard et al. (1984) found that vision loss was associated with depression, but only among those with a low degree of social support; among those with high support, no correlation emerged. Overall, the attitudes, behaviors, and perceptions of family members appear to play a significant role in the overall adjustment of older visually impaired persons (Large, 1982; Morrison, 1982).

Based upon this growing body of evidence, there has been an increasing recognition of the critical need to include the family as an active member of the rehabilitation team, as well as an increasing awareness that the family has unique needs that must be addressed in addition to their role as "partner" and adjunct in the rehabilitation process for the older adult (see Chapter 6; Betts, 1990; Brummel-Smith, 1988, 1992; Cook & Ferritor, 1985; Kelly & Lambert, 1992; Kemp, 1990; Smith & Messikomer, 1988; Youngblood & Hines, 1992).

Although the evidence of need is obvious, few rehabilitation facilities have treatment programs specifically targeted to family members (Smith & Messikomer, 1988). Given the dearth of programs, it is not surprising that there is also limited evidence on the effectiveness of family intervention programs relative to either patient or family functioning.

Overall, the current state of the art in rehabilitation and aging provides ample clinical examples but limited empirically based evidence that families, for better or worse, are both influenced by and influential in the rehabilitation process and outcomes for older adults. More extensive experience with family intervention models and careful evaluation of their results is critically needed as we move forward with the inclusion of family members in the rehabilitation process. As Kelly & Lambert (1992) emphasize, "although the literature is replete with anecdotal reports describing persons who have, do, or will benefit from specific family rehabilitation strategies, there are few systematic well-controlled (demonstration) studies."

Comorbidity Among Elders with Visual Impairments

Attention to general health status and concurrent impairments is important in any study addressing older adults. Vision impairment is only one of many age-related impairments affecting the elderly. In fact, epidemiological data suggest that at least two-thirds of all visually impaired older persons experience at least one (and more likely two or more) concurrent health conditions (Kirchner, 1985); and the likelihood of comorbidity obviously increases as the age of the elder increases. Therefore, we must remember that vision loss can neither be treated nor studied in isolation. Although vision is often a contributor to the overall disability of the older person, it is rarely the sole impairment. Not only do we need to isolate the independent influence of vision impairment on functional and psychological status, but we also need to better understand how it interacts with other impairments to affect overall functional status and quality of life.

Of particular interest is the experience of a dual sensory impairment in later life. Although there is an emerging literature regarding the profound functional and psychological consequences of either a vision or hearing impairment in later life, the special circumstances of dual sensory impaired elderly (i.e., concurrent age-related impairment of vision and hearing) have been largely ignored in the research literature. Yet, given that vision and hearing impairments are among the most common chronic conditions of later life that increase in prevalence with advanced age, coupled with the aging of the population, the numbers of older people experiencing a concurrent age-related loss in both vision and hearing can be expected to grow substantially. Even current estimates of the prevalence of dual sensory impairments among the elderly range as high as 18 percent (Horowitz & Stuen, 1991). Yet, this is a subgroup of the elderly that has long been ignored by both the research and the service community and its members truly represent the "unseen and unheard" among the larger population of older persons.

For example, only limited and contradictory evidence exists regarding the effects of concurrent age-related losses in both hearing and vision on functional disability. In a cross-sectional study of 1,191 community-based elders ages 70 to 75 in Italy, Appollonio, Carabellese, Frattola, and Trabucchi (1995) found that a dual sensory impairment did not lead to additional deterioration of ADL and IADL scores over the presence of a single sensory deficit in either hearing or vision. However, in a sample of more than 1,400 elders with baseline and 1-year follow-up data, LaForge et al. (1992) report that, although hearing impairment was not related to functional decline, elders with dual sensory impairments had a 40 percent greater risk of functional decline over those with impairments in vision only. These preliminary findings regarding the impact of dual sensory impairment are limited to cross-sectional or short-term follow-up analyses only, and again highlight the need for a more systematic study of the long-term consequences of dual sensory impairment, utilizing multiple and long-term follow-ups.

Thus, although it has been suggested from clinical literature that ". . . the presence of two sensory losses increases the functional significance of each one; . . . a loss which by standard measures might be considered mild or even inconsequential may be substantially limiting when combined with a loss of the other major sense" (Luey, Belser, & Glass, 1989), little data exist to either support or refute this hypothesis. This gap in the knowledge base has severely limited the ability to plan effective service interventions to address the needs of the growing numbers of elders who will experience concurrent age-related vision and hearing impairments in later life.

Subjective Appraisals of Vision Loss

There is emerging evidence that the loss of vision is perceived as more disabling and is more feared than other physical impairments (The Lighthouse Inc., 1995). Historically, and at the most irrational level, blindness has been associated with punishment for sin, a view reflected in biblical, mythological, and Shakespearian literature (Monbeck, 1975). One public opinion poll found that blindness ranks fourth, following only AIDS, cancer, and Alzheimer's disease, as the health condition most feared by Americans of all ages, primarily because of its association with complete helplessness and dependency (National Society for the Prevention of Blindness, 1984–85).

Elders who become visually impaired in later life have often internalized this devaluating orientation, which in turn influences the subjective meaning they ascribe to both the visual impairment itself and the functional limitations associated with the vision impairment. In fact, in a study of 11 common chronic conditions of later life, vision impairment emerged as one of only three conditions that independently predicted depression when demographics, social support, and all other health conditions were held constant; this finding suggests that vision loss is, in fact or perception, more functionally and emotionally debilitating than many other age-related health problems (Bazargan & Hamm-Baugh, 1995).

Thus, the onset of a visual impairment in later life may engender a unique set of fears and reactions among older persons. For example, the older person who is experiencing problems in mobility attributable to visual impairment may have a totally different subjective experience of this limitation than the older person with arthritis who is experiencing a similar set of functional mobility problems. Furthermore, if vision loss is something to be feared, it may also be something to be denied, to self and to others, for as long as possible. In sum, subjective appraisals of the vision loss may have implications for compensatory efforts, including help-seeking behaviors, and ultimately adaptation to the visual impairment. Again, however, little data are available to support or refute these hypotheses. Given the implications for better understanding and facilitating the pathways by which older people do seek rehabilitation services, research into the significance ascribed to vision loss in later life, relative to other age-related conditions, is another important direction for future research.

Peer Support Groups

A growing clinical and empirical literature supports the positive influence of peer support groups for a variety of health conditions across age groups (see, e.g., Koop, 1992; Madara & Meese, 1988; Reisman & Carroll, 1995). However, little of this research has focused on peer support groups for older adults with visual impairments. This lack of research attention is not because such groups are rare. In fact, a national survey conducted by The Lighthouse Inc. identified more than 400 peer support groups serving visually impaired adults, the vast majority of which were affiliated with a vision rehabilitation organization. Focus group interviews conducted as part of this survey yielded qualitative data supporting the value the members placed on the groups in helping them overcome hopelessness and generally adapt to their vision loss (Stuen, 1993). Yet, there is not one single systematic empirical study of the effectiveness of peer support groups as either a single resource or as part of a more comprehensive vision rehabilitation program. Some very basic questions remain unexplored, such as:

What are the characteristics of older adults who are most likely to participate in support groups? At what stage in the experience of vision loss are peer support groups most effective? And at what stage in the rehabilitation process (prior, during, or after service) is this intervention most beneficial in terms of both functional and psychosocial outcomes?

Furthermore, peer support groups can and do take many forms in composition, format, as well as mode of delivery. For example, groups can be disease specific or not; they can be solely peer-led or co-led by a professional; groups may consist only of older adults who are visually impaired or may include family members as well. Advances in technology have provided alternatives to face-to-face meetings, for example, via telephone or through the Internet. Comparative studies of various types of peer support groups would add significantly to the knowledge base needed to plan services that effectively and efficiently meet the needs of the growing numbers of older persons with vision impairments.

Age, Gender, and Ethnic Differences

Epidemiological data clearly document the relationship between increasing age and the experience of vision impairment (see, e.g., Branch et al., 1989; Havlik, 1986; Salive et al., 1992; Tielsch, Sommer, Witt, Katz, & Royall, 1990). Race and socioeconomic status have also been found to be strongly and independently associated with the experience of vision impairment, with African-Americans and those with lower levels of income and education evidencing significantly higher rates of impairment (Grey, Burns-Cox, & Hughes, 1989; Klein, Klein, Jensen, Moss, & Cruickshanks, 1994; Seddon, 1991; Sommer et al., 1991; Salive et al., 1992; Tielsch et al., 1990, 1991). On the other hand, most epidemiological studies show no gender difference in the overall prevalence of vision impairment among the elderly (see, e.g., Branch et al., 1989; Tielsch, Javitt, Coleman, Katz, & Sommer, 1995; Verbrugge & Patrick, 1995). However, in terms of the psychosocial aspects of vision loss and vision rehabilitation, relatively little data are available that address age, gender, and racial or ethnic differences.

It is important to remember that the elderly are not a homogeneous group and that many cohorts, each with different histories and life experiences, are represented within the "65 and older" population. Although chronological age has been found to be a powerful predictor of many outcome variables in gerontological research, in research about vision and aging it is important to consider not only current age, but age at onset of the vision problems as well.

It may be hypothesized that, because vision loss has become an "expected" condition of later life, it will be less stressful and better tolerated by the oldest old, who will define it as an "on-time" event in their lives. The oldest old will also be able to draw upon the array of coping strategies developed over time to deal with age-related disabilities. In fact, some researchers have suggested that the relationship between disability and depression may actually become weaker with advancing age; that is, older age brings an increasing ability to cope with adversity (Gurland, Wilder, & Berkman, 1988). In contrast, for the younger elderly, who are less likely to have experienced other concurrent losses associated with aging, the onset of a vision problem often represents the first negative age-related event. It may therefore be defined as "off-time" in terms of its occurrence in the life cycle, and thus engender heightened stress and, in turn, negatively influence adaptation.

A competing hypothesis regarding the effect of age proposes a negative relationship between more successful adaptation and age at onset. That is, a vision loss will represent a more severe stress for the oldest old, owing to both the multiple health conditions they are likely to experience and the diminishing of social support resources. Furthermore, because they grew up and grew old with very different conceptions of aging, the oldest-old cohort may be more likely to accept disability as a "normal" consequence of aging rather than to actively pursue compensatory interventions. Younger elderly people, however, may be more action oriented. They may be more likely to reject the stereotype that equates age with disability. As a result, the younger elderly may be able to bring greater emotional and physical resources to the adaptation process and may be more likely to seek the help needed to help them compensate for functional losses.

Each of these scenarios regarding the relationship between age and adaptation to vision impairment remains a hypothesis, however. The influence of age and age at onset of vision loss, within the context of other social and psychological factors, requires further research.

Similarly, little is known about the differences between older men and women in terms of processes of adaptation to the vision impairment and the relative effectiveness of rehabilitation interventions. A body of research in the gerontological literature supports the existence of significant gender differences in many aspects of aging. For example, women tend to be able to draw on a larger array of social supports in the family and friendship networks (see, e.g., Wright, 1989), which might positively influence adaptation to a vision disability. On the other hand, empirical evidence indicates that women experience depression about twice as frequently as men (see Culbertson, 1997 for review), and thus would appear to be at greater risk of poorer adaptation to a vision impairment as compared to men. Some studies among visually impaired elders have documented significantly higher depressive symptoms in women than in men (Horowitz et al., 1994; Reinhardt, 1996), whereas others have failed to find such gender differences in depression (e.g., Hersen et al., 1995; Shmuely-Dulitzki, Rovner, & Zisselman, 1995). Clearly, the relationship between gender and the processes and outcomes of adaptation is an area that also requires future research.

Finally, most studies in the psychosocial aspects of vision and aging, as well as in outcomes of rehabilitation services, have been limited by the failure to include sufficient numbers of racial or ethnic minorities which would permit analyses to identify differences in experiences with vision impairment. It is known that there are significant variations in how different ethnic and racial groups react to a disability (i.e., the subjective appraisal), how they view the family's role vis-à-vis disabled relatives, as well as the extent to which they are able or willing to access formal services, such as vision rehabilitation, to deal with the disabling effect of age-related impairments. To develop culturally relevant outreach and service strategies, future research in aging and vision needs to give greater attention to ethnic differences and ensure any new disability questions reflect variations in ethnic/cultural understanding of disability (National Council on Disability, 1998).

CONCLUSION

This chapter has attempted to identify critical directions for future research in aging, vision impairment, and vision rehabilitation. The emphasis has been on highlighting the unknown. Although it is clear that the field remains at the early stages of developing an empirical knowledge base, the future of research in aging and vision should be considered promising. Recently published research studies in the field have increased not only in number but also in quality. Furthermore, this research can be found in both the vision rehabilitation literature and in the mainstream of the gerontological research literature, as more gerontologists are becoming interested in issues related to sensory loss in later life and as vision rehabilitation researchers are increasingly addressing questions specific to the elderly. However, rather than continuing in two parallel but distinct directions, the challenge now is to form a partnership between the two fields. Only by bringing together the unique perspectives of each discipline will it be possible to optimize the development of a conceptually relevant and empirically based body of knowledge critically needed to provide the foundation for the design and delivery of effective interventions for elders with age-related vision loss.

There is no doubt that a full agenda faces researchers, and one that will only increase in scope as more sophisticated questions are raised relevant to understanding the experience of vision loss in later life. It is also a research agenda that will increase in importance with the projected growth and aging of the older population, resulting in increasing numbers of elders affected by age-related vision loss. Yet, it is important to bear in mind that the cohorts of older people are continuously changing. In general, demographic projections indicate that the elderly of the future will be better educated, and will have grown up and grown older in a society with more positive attitudes and approaches toward both aging and disability. In all probability, the future elderly will evidence more aggressive approaches to accessing appropriate medical and rehabilitation services. They will be less likely to accept any age-related loss as "normal." Therefore, the development of a research agenda is an ongoing process and one that must be continuously reevaluated and updated in response to changing times and changing cohorts of the elderly.

REFERENCES

Aneshensel, C. S., Pearlin, L. I., Mullan J. T., Zarit, S. H., & Whitlatch, C. J. (1995). *Profiles in caregiving: The unexpected career.* San Diego, CA: Academic Press.

Appollonio, I., Carabellese, C. Magni, E., Frattola, L., & Trabucchi, M. (1995). Sensory impairments and mortality in an elderly community population: A six-year follow-up study. *Age and Aging, 24,* 3–36.

Bazargan, M., & Hamm-Baugh, V. P. (1995). The relationship between chronic illness and depression in a community of urban black elderly persons. *Journal of Gerontology: Social Sciences, 50B,* S119–S127.

Becker, G., & Kaufman, S. (1988). Old age, rehabilitation and research: A review of the issues. *The Gerontologist, 28,* 459–468.

Betts, H. B. (1990). Rehabilitation and the elderly: A psychiatrist's view. In S. J. Brody & L. G. Pawlson (Eds.), *Aging and rehabilitation II: The state of the practice.* New York: Springer, pp. 30–40.

Biegel, D. E., & Blum, A. (1990). *Aging and caregiving: Theory, research and practice.* Newbury Park, CA: Sage.

Biegel, D. E., Sales, E., & Schultz, R. (1991). *Family caregiving in chronic illness.* Newbury Park, CA: Sage.

Branch, L. G., Horowitz, A., & Carr, C. (1989). The implications for everyday life of incident reported visual decline among people over age 65 living in the community. *The Gerontologist, 29,* 359–365.

Brody, E. M. (1985). Parent care as a normative family stress. *The Gerontologist, 25,* 19–29.

Brody, E. M. (1986). Informal support systems in the rehabilitation of the disabled elderly. In S. J. Brody & G. E. Ruff (Eds.), *Aging and rehabilitation: Advances in the state of the art.* New York: Springer, pp. 87–103.

Brummel-Smith, K. (1988). Family science and geriatric rehabilitation. *Topics in Geriatric Rehabilitation, 4,* 1–7.

Brummel-Smith, K. (1992). Geriatric rehabilitation. *Generations, XVI,* 27–30.

Cantor, M., & Little, V. (1985). Aging and social care. In R. H. Binstock & E. Shanas (Eds.), *Handbook of aging and the social sciences* (2nd ed.). New York: Van Nostrand Reinhold.

Carabellese, C., Appollonio, I., Rozzini, R., Bianchetti, A., Frisoni, G. B., Frattola, L., & Trabucchi, M. (1993). Sensory impairment and quality of life in a community elderly population. *Journal of the American Geriatrics Society, 41,* 401–407.

Cook, G. S. & Ferritor, D. (1985). The family: A potential resource in the provision of rehabilitation services. *Journal of Rehabilitation Counseling, 16,* 52–53.

Crews, J. E. (1991). Measuring rehabilitation outcomes and the public policies of aging and blindness. In N. Weber (Ed.), *Vision and aging: Issues in social work practice.* New York: Haworth, pp. 137–151.

Crews, J. E., & Frey, W. D. (1993). Family concerns and older people who are blind. *Journal of Visual Impairment & Blindness, 87,* 6–11.

Crews, J. E., & Long, R. G. (1997). Conceptual and methodological issues in rehabilitation outcomes for adults who are visually impaired. *Journal of Visual Impairment & Blindness, 91,* 117–130.

Culbertson, F. M. (1997). Depression and gender: An international review. *American Psychologist, 52,* 25–31.

Cummings, S. R., Phillips, S. L., Wheat, M. E., Black, D., Goosby, E., Wlodarczyk, D., Trafton, P., Jergesen, H., Winograd, C. H., & Hulley, S. B. (1988). Recovery of function after hip fracture: The role of social supports. *Journal of the Gerontological Society, 36,* 801–808.

Dodds, A. G., Bailey, P., Pearson, A., & Yates, L. (1991). Psychological factors in acquired visual impairment: The development of a scale of adjustment. *Journal of Visual Impairment & Blindness, 85*(7), 306–310.

Dodds, A., Ferguson, E., Ng, L., Flannigan, H., Hawes, G., & Yates, L. (1994). The concept of adjustment: A structural model. *Journal of Visual Impairment & Blindness, 88*(6), 487–497.

Dodds, A. G., Flannigan, H., & Ng, L. (1993). The Nottingham Adjustment Scale: A validation study. *International Journal of Rehabilitation Research, 16,* 177–184.

Dumas, A., & Sadowsky, A. D. (1984). A family training program for adventitiously blinded and low vision veterans. *Journal of Visual Impairment & Blindness, 78,* 473–478.

Ehmer, M. N., & Needham, W. E. (1979). *The beliefs about blindness scale.* New Haven, CT: Authors.

Emerson, D. L. (1981). Fading loss of vision: The response of adults to visual impairments. *Journal of Visual Impairment & Blindness, 75,* 41–45.

Evans, R. L., Bishop, D. S., Matlock, A. L., Stranahan, S., Smith, G., & Halar, E. (1987). Family interaction and treatment adherence after stroke. *Archives of Physical Medicine and Rehabilitation, 68,* 513–517.

Fitting, E. A. (1954). *Evaluation of adjustment to blindness.* New York: American Foundation for the Blind.

Ford, A. B., Folmar, S. J., Salmon, R. B., Medalie, J. H., Roy, A. W., & Galazka, S. S. (1988). Health and function in the old and very old. *Journal of the American Geriatrics Society, 36,* 187–197.

Freedman, V. A., Berkman, L. F., Rapp, S. R. & Ostfeld, A. M. (1994). Family networks: Predictors of nursing home entry. *American Journal of Public Health, 84,* 843–845.

Furner, S. E., Rudberg, M. A., & Cassel, C. K. (1995). Medical conditions differentially affect the development of IADL disability: Implications for medical care and research. *The Gerontologist, 35*(4), 444–450.

George, L., & Gwyther, L. P. (1986). Caregiver well-being: A multidimensional examination of family caregivers of demented adults. *The Gerontologist, 26,* 253–259.

Golden, R. R., Teresi, J. A., & Gurland, B. J. (1984). Development of indicator scales for the comprehensive assessment and referral evaluation (CARE) interview schedule. *Journal of Gerontology, 39*(2), 138–146.

Goodman, C. R., Horowitz, A., Reinhardt, J. P., & Bird, B. (1996). Comparisons of older adult and family perceptions of vision impairment. Poster presented at the Annual Scientific Meeting of the Gerontological Society of America, Washington, DC.

Grey, R. H. B., Burns-Cox, C. J., & Hughes, A. (1989). Blind and partial sight registration in Avon. *British Journal of Ophthalmology, 79,* 99–104.

Grieg, D. E., West, M. I., & Overbury, O. (1986). Successful use of low vision aids: Visual and psychological factors. *Journal of Visual Impairment & Blindness, 80,* 985–988.

Gurland, B., Wilder, D. E., & Berkman, C. (1988). Depression and disability in the elderly: Reciprocal relations and changes with age. *International Journal of Geriatric Psychiatry, 3,* 163–179.

Hanley, R. J., Alecxih, L. M., Wiener, J. M., & Kennell, D. L. (1990). Predicting elderly nursing home admissions: Results from the 1982–1984 National Long-Term Care Survey. *Research in Aging, 12,* 199–228.

Havlik, R. J. (1986). *Aging in the eighties: Impaired senses for sound and light in persons age 65 years and over.* NCHS, Advance Data Vital and Health Statistics of the National Center for Health Statistics, No. 125.

Heinemann, A. W., Colorez, A., Frank, S., & Taylor, D. (1988). Leisure activity participation of elderly individuals with low vision. *The Gerontologist, 2,* 181–184.

Hersen, M., Kabacoff, R. I., Van Hasselt, V. B., Null, J. A., Ryan, C. F., Melton, M. A., & Segal, D. L. (1995). Assertiveness, depression and social support in older visually impaired adults. *Journal of Visual Impairment & Blindness, 89,* 524–530.

Horowitz, A. (1985). Caregiving to the frail elderly. In M. P. Lawton & G. Maddox (Eds.), *Annual review of geriatrics and gerontology.* New York: Springer.

Horowitz, A., Goodman, C. R., & Reinhardt, J. P. (1998). *Vision rehabilitation and family services: Maximizing functional and psychosocial status for both older visually impaired adults and their families: Part II. The research evaluation.* Final report submitted to the AARP Andrus Foundation. New York: The Lighthouse Inc., Arlene R. Gordon Research Institute.

Horowitz, A., Leonard, R., & Reinhardt, J. P. (1996). *Adaptive skills training program: Year 1 evaluation report.* New York: The Lighthouse Inc., Arlene R. Gordon Research Institute.

Horowitz, A., Leonard, R., & Reinhardt, J. P. (1997a). *Adaptive skills training program: Year 2 evaluation report.* New York: The Lighthouse Inc., Arlene R. Gordon Research Institute.

Horowitz, A., Leonard, R., & Reinhardt, J. P. (1997b). *Integrated rehabilitation services for the elderly: Year 1 evaluation report.* New York: The Lighthouse Inc., Arlene R. Gordon Research Institute.

Horowitz, A., & Reinhardt, J. P. (1992). *Assessing adaptation to age-related vision loss.* New York: The Lighthouse Research Institute.

Horowitz, A., & Reinhardt, J. P. (1998). Development of the adaptation to age-related vision loss scale. *Journal of Visual Impairment & Blindness, 92,* 30–41.

Horowitz, A., & Reinhardt, J. P. (in press). Mental health issues in visual impairment: Research in depression, disability, and rehabilitation. In B. Silverstone, M. Lang, B. Rosenthal, & E. Faye (Eds.), *The Lighthouse handbook on vision impairment and vision rehabilitation.* New York: Oxford University Press.

Horowitz, A., Reinhardt, J. P., McInerney, R., & Balistreri, E. (1994). *Age-related vision loss: Factors associated with adaptation to chronic impairment over time.* Final report submitted to the AARP-Andrus Foundation. New York: The Lighthouse Inc.

Horowitz, A., & Stuen, C. (1991). The prevalence and correlation of concurrent vision and hearing impairment among the elderly. Paper presented at the Annual Scientific Meeting of the Gerontological Society of America.

Kaufman, R., Albright, L., & Wagner, C. (1987). Rehabilitation outcomes after hip fracture in persons 90 years old and older. *Archives of Physical and Medical rehabilitation, 68,* 369–671.

Kelly, S. D. M., & Lambert, S. S. (1992). Family support in rehabilitation: A review of research 1980–1990. *Rehabilitation Counseling Bulletin, 36,* 98–119.

Kemp, B. (1990). The psychosocial context of geriatric rehabilitation. In B. Kemp, K. Brummel-Smith, & J. W. Ramsdell (Eds.), *Geriatric Rehabilitation.* Boston: College-Hill Press, pp. 41–57.

Kirchner, C. (1985). *Data on blindness and visual impairment in the United States.* New York: American Foundation for the Blind.

Kirchner, C. (in press). Methodological strategies and issues in social research on visual impairment and rehabilitation. In B. Silverstone, M. Lang, B. Rosenthal, E. Faye (Eds.), *The Lighthouse handbook on vision impairment and vision rehabilitation.* New York: Oxford University Press.

Klein, R., Klein, B. E., Jensen, S. C., Moss, S. E., & Cruickshanks, K. J. (1994). The relation of socioeconomic factors to age-related cataract, maculopathy, and impaired vision: The Beaver Dam Eye Study. *Ophthalmology, 101*, 1969–1970.

Koop, C. E. (1992). Sharing solutions keynote address. *Aging & Vision News, 4* (2), 1–11.

LaForge, R. G., Spector, W. D., & Sternberg, J. (1992). The relationship of vision and hearing impairment to one-year mortality and functional decline. *Journal of Aging and Health, 4*, 126–148.

Large, T. (1982). Effects of attitudes upon the blind: A re-examination. *Journal of Rehabilitation, 48*, 33–34, 45.

Lazarus, R. S., & DeLongis, A. (1983). Psychological stress and coping in aging. *American Psychologist, 31*, 245–254.

Lazarus, R. S., & Folkman, S. (1984). *Stress, appraisal and coping.* New York: Springer.

Lee, D., Gomez-Marin, O., & Lam, B. (1996). Depressive symptoms and visual acuity in Hispanic adult. Paper presented at the Annual Scientific Meeting of the Gerontological Society of America, Washington, DC; November, 1996.

The Lighthouse Inc. (1995). *The Lighthouse National Survey on Vision Loss: The experiences, attitudes, and knowledge of middle-aged and older Americans.* New York: The Lighthouse Inc.

Long, R. G., Crews, J. E., & Mancil, R. (1995). *Final report: Functional independence measure for blind adults (Project N. C699-RA).* Decatur, Georgia: Rehabilitation Research and Development Center, VA Medical Center–Atlanta.

Luey, H. S., Belser, D., & Glass, L. (1989). *Beyond refuge: Coping with losses in vision and hearing.* (1989). University of California, San Francisco, Center on Deafness. Helen Keller Center for Deaf-Blind Youth and Adults.

Lukoff, I. F., & Whiteman, M. (1970). *The social sources of adjustment to blindness.* New York: American Foundation for the Blind Press.

Madara, E. J., & Meese A. (1988) *The self-help sourcebook.* Denville, New Jersey: St. Clare's-Riverside Medical Center.

McFall, S., & Miller, B. H. (1992). Caregiver burden and nursing home admission of frail elderly persons. *Journal of Gerontology, 47*, S73–S79.

Monbeck, M. E. (1975). *The meaning of blindness.* London: Indiana University Press.

Moore, J. E. (1984). Impact of family attitudes toward blindness/vision impairment on the rehabilitation process. *Journal of Blindness & Visual Impairment, 78*, 100–106.

Mor, V., Murphy, J., Masterson-Allen, S., Willey, G., Razmpour, A., Jackson, M. E., Greer, D., & Katz, S. (1989). Risk of functional decline among well elders. *Journal of Clinical Epidemiology, 42*, 895–904.

National Council on Disability (1998). *Reorienting disability research.* Washington DC: National Council on Disability.

National Eye Institute. (1996). *Visual Functioning Questionnaire-25 (VFQ-25).* Washington, DC: National Eye Institute.

National Society for the Prevention of Blindness. (1984–85). Survey '84: Attitudes towards blindness prevention. *Sight-Saving, 53,* 14–17.

Needham, W. E., & Ehmer, M. N. (1980). Irrational thinking and adjustment to vision loss. *Journal of Visual Impairment and Blindness, 74,* 57–61.

Oppegard, K., Hansson, R. O., Morgan, T., Indart, M., Crutcher, M., & Hampton, P. (1984). Sensory loss, family support, and adjustment among the elderly. *The Journal of Social Psychology, 123,* 291–292.

Osterweil, D. (1990). Geriatric rehabilitation in the long-term care institutional setting. In B. Kemp, K. Brummel-Smith, & J. W. Ramsdell (Eds.), *Geriatric rehabilitation.* Boston: College-Hill Press, pp. 347–356.

Reinhardt, J. P. (1996). Importance of friendship and family support in adaptation to chronic vision impairment. *Journal of Gerontology: Psychological Sciences, 51B,* P268–P278.

Reissman, F., & Carroll, D. (1995). *Redefining self-help.* San Francisco: Jossey-Bass.

Ringering, L., & Amaral, P. (in press). The role of psychosocial factors in adaptation to visual impairment and rehabilitation outcomes for adults and older adults. In B. Silverstone, M. Lang, B. Rosenthal, & E. Faye (Eds.), *The Lighthouse handbook on vision impairment and vision rehabilitation.* New York: Oxford University Press.

Roberto, K. A. (1992). Elderly women with hip fractures: Functional and psychosocial correlates of recovery. *Journal of Women and Aging, 4,* 3–20.

Rosenbloom, A. A., & Goodrich, G. L. (1997). Low vision rehabilitation: Emerging research and development challenges. Paper presented at the Asian Pacific Optometric Conference, Seoul, Korea.

Salive, M. E., Guralnik, J., Christen, W., Glynn, R. J., Colsher, P., & Ostfeld, A. M. (1992). Functional blindness and visual impairment in older adults from three communities. *Ophthalmology, 99,* 1840–1847.

Salive, M. E., Guralnik, J., Glynn, R. J., Christen, W., Wallace, R. B., & Ostfeld, A. M. (1994). Association of visual impairment with mobility and physical function. *Journal of the American Geriatrics Society, 42,* 287–292.

Schulz, R., Visintainer, P., & Williamson, G. M. (1990). Psychiatric and physical morbidity effects of caregiving. *Journal of Gerontology: Psychological Sciences, 45,* 181–191.

Seddon, J. M. (1991). The differential burden of blindness in the United States. *New England Journal of Medicine, 325,* 1422–1440.

Shmuely-Dulitzki, Y., Rovner, B. W., & Zisselman, P. (1995). The impact of depression on functioning in elderly patients with low vision. *The American Journal of Geriatric Psychiatry, 3*(4), 325–329.

Silverstone, B. M. (1984). Social aspects of rehabilitation. In T. F. Williams (Ed.), *Rehabilitation in the aging*. New York: Raven Press, pp. 59–79.

Silverstone, B. M. (1998). A grain of salt. Paper presented at the Annual Meeting of the American Society on Aging. San Francisco, California.

Smith, V. J., & Messikomer, C. M. (1988). A role for the family in geriatric rehabilitation. *Topics in Geriatric Rehabilitation, 4*, 8–15.

Sommer, A., Tielsch, J. M., Ketz, J., Quigley, H. A., Gottsch, J. D., Javitt, J. C., Martone, J. F., Royall, R. M., Witt, K. A., & Ezrine, S. (1991). Racial differences in the cause specific prevalence of blindness's in East Baltimore. *New England Journal of Medicine, 325*,1412–1417.

Stone, R., Cafferata, G. L., & Sangl, J. (1987). Caregivers of the frail elderly: A national profile. *The Gerontologist, 27*, 616–626.

Stuen, C. (1993). Self help/mutual aid support groups for visually impaired older adults. Proceedings of the Second National Conference: The Challenge to Independence. New York: Helen Keller National Center.

Thomas, T., & Stevens, R. (1974). Social effects of fractures of the femur. *British Medical Journal, 3*, 456–458.

Tielsch, J. M., Javitt, J. C., Coleman, A., Katz, J. & Sommer, A. (1995). The prevalence of blindness and visual impairment among nursing home residents in Baltimore. *The New England Journal of Medicine, 332*, 1205–1209.

Tielsch, J. M., Sommer, A., Katz, J., Quigley, H., Ezrine, S., & the Baltimore Eye Survey Research Group. (1991). Socioeconomic status and visual impairment among urban Americans. *Archives of Ophthalmology, 109*, 637–641.

Tielsch, J. M., Sommer, A., Witt, K., Katz, J., & Royall, R. M. (1990). Blindness and visual impairment in an American urban population: The Baltimore Eye Survey. *Archives of Ophthalmology, 108*, 286–290.

Verbruge, L. M., & Patrick, D. L. (1995). Seven chronic conditions: Their impact on US adults' activity levels and use of medical services. *American Journal of Public Health, 85*(2), 173–182.

Wahl, H.-W., & Oswald, F. (in press). The person/environment perspective of visual impairment. In B. Silverstone, M. Lang, B. Rosenthal, & E. Faye (Eds.), *The Lighthouse handbook on vision impairment and vision rehabilitation*. New York: Oxford University Press.

Warren, M., & Lampert, J. (1994). Considerations in addressing the daily living needs in older persons with low vision. *Ophthalmology Clinics of North America, 7*(2), 187–195.

Wright, P. H. (1989). Gender differences in adults' same and cross-gender friendships. In R. G. Adams & R. Blieszner (Eds.), *Older adults friendship: Structure and process*. Newbury Park, CA: Sage, pp. 197–221.

Youngblood, N. M., & Hines, J. (1992). The influence of the family's perception of disability on rehabilitation outcomes. *Rehabilitation Nursing, 17*(6), 323–326.

Index

A

Activities of daily living (ADL)
  adaptations to, 27
  age and impairment, 6
  instrumental ADLs, 42, 133
  rehabilitation for, 69
  and type of impairment, 26, 42
  and vision loss, 40, 42, 133
Adaptation to Age-Related Vision
    Loss (AVL) scale, 232
Adaptation to vision loss, 228–234
  longitudinal studies, 233–234
  measurement of, 232–233
  and rehabilitation outcomes, 234–238
  samples studied, 233–234
  and social support, 231
  stress and coping model for, 230–231
Administration on Aging, projects
    of, 200–201
African Americans
  in aging population, 7
  and diabetic retinopathy, 60
  and glaucoma, 60
Ageism
  meaning of, 78
  myths about aging, 110
Age-related macular degeneration,
    33, 62–63, 93–94

dry type, 93
  management of, 94
  nature of, 62–63, 93–94
  vision loss from, 63, 93–94
  wet type, 93
Aging
  age span classification, 6
  chronic conditions of, 27, 116, 122
  and disability, 26–32
  and diversity, 25
  and frailty, 117–120
  and gender, 7
  geriatric syndromes, types of,
    122–126
  and income, 7–8, 10
  and learning style, 127
  life expectancy, extension of, 15–16, 23
  marginalized societal status of,
    186–189
  medicalization of, 195–197
  and national economic growth,
    12–13
  and neurological functions, 116
  and normal visual changes, 87,
    115
  and physiological changes, 114–116
  and policy dilemmas, 23–26
  population trends, 5–8, 23–26
  public attitude toward, 32

and public policy, 8–11, 44–46, 183–206
and social class, 15
vision-related issues and, 18–19, 22–23
Aging network
members of, 212
role of, 79–80, 189
Aging and visual impairment
adaptation, research on, 228–234
age and adaptation to vision loss, 246–247
age range and impairment, 5–6, 38
relationship between, 18–19
and family, 161–164
implications of, 56–57
population estimates, 32–39, 59–60, 86–87
prevalence of, 27
psychosocial effects of, 67–69
secondary conditions, 39–42
underlying conditions, 136
See also Visual conditions
Alzheimer's disease, 116
incidence of, 123
American Foundation for the Blind, 215
Americans with Disabilities Act, 77
Antidepressants, 124–125, 147
Aqueous humor, function of, 92
Area Agencies on Aging (AAAs), 223
Area Planning and Service Committee (APSC), 203, 205
Arthritis, 27
Association for Education and Rehabilitation of the Blind and Visually Impaired, 218
Atherosclerosis, 27

B

Baby boom, 15
and the elderly population, 23
and vision loss, 59
Balance problems, 96
causes of, 125
Baltimore Nursing Home Eye Survey, 35, 38
Biopsychosocial perspective, 134–135
Blindness
among older people, 5
ICD classification, 89
legal, definition of, 88
Blind spots, 95
Bureau of the Census, Survey of Income and Program Participation (SIPP), 35, 37
Bureau of Health Professionals, 202

C

Cardiovascular system, and aging, 114
Cataracts, 33, 38, 65–66, 91
nature of, 65, 91
prevalence among older people, 27
treatment of, 65–66, 91
Cerebrovascular disease, prevalence among older people, 27
Certification, vision practitioners, 218
Chronic bronchitis, prevalence among older people, 27
Chronic sinusitis, prevalence among older people, 27
Civil rights movement, 8–9
Closed-angle glaucoma, nature of, 63, 93
Closed-circuit television systems (CCTVs), 98, 99, 219
Coalitions, between the aging and disability fields, 198–201
Cognitive-behavioral therapy, for depression, 146–147
Cognitive impairment, 124

Community-based service, vision rehabilitation as, 76
Co-morbidity, research on, 241–243
Comprehensive Outpatient Rehabilitation Facility (CORF), 221
Consumers
  consumer empowerment, 216–217
  consumer support groups, 214–215
Cornea, function of, 88
Crowding phenomenon, 95

D

Dark adaptation, 87, 95–96
Defined-contribution plans, 8
Delirium, causes of, 124
Dementia, 38
  Alzheimer's disease, 123
  and medical rehabilitation, 124
Demographics
  aging and visual impairment estimates, 32–39, 59–60, 86–87
  baby boomers, 15–16, 23
  and trends in aging, 5–8, 23–26, 61–62
Denial, of vision loss, 163
Depression, 39, 42, 137, 142–147
  assessment of, 145–146
  biochemical factors, 144–145
  medical intervention for, 124–125, 147
  and mortality, 143
  predisposing factors, 144
  psychotherapy for, 146–147
  signs of, 124, 142
  and social support, 145
  stress and coping model of, 143–144
Desyrel, 147
Developmental disabilities, 189–190
  forms of, 190
Diabetes, 33, 137

prevalence among older people, 27
and visual impairment. *See* Diabetic retinopathy
Diabetic retinopathy, 64–65, 91–92
  and ethnic minorities, 60, 65
  management of, 64, 92
  nature of, 64
Disability, definition of, 134
Disability and aging, 26–32
  chronic conditions, listing of, 27
  and life expectancy, 29–30
  rates of disability, 27–28
Disability glare, 100
Discomfort glare, 100
Driving, 67
Dry type, age-related macular degeneration, 93
Dual sensory impairment, 242–243
Dysfunction, common causes of, 135

E

Educational level, and health status, 28
Emphysema, prevalence among older people, 27
Entitlements, 14
Ethnic minorities
  and aging, 25
  and diabetic retinopathy, 60, 65
  and vision loss, 60, 247
Exercise, 120–122
  benefits of, 41, 120
  and client compliance, 120
  and facors affecting, 121
  strength training, 121
Eye, structures of, 88, 90–91

F

Falls, 39, 125
Family
  burdened family style, 150

as caregiver, 192–195
caregiver stress, 158–159
conflicted family style, 150
dysfunctional styles, 150
family support, effects on
    disabled person, 159–160
healthy family style, 150
hierarchical support role, 158
members living together, 157–158
rating system for, 149
research on caregivers, 239–241
and vision loss, 68–69, 161–164
women as caregivers, 193
Family Futures Training Project, 200
Family-oriented rehabilitation, 138–
    139, 141, 155–157, 159–160,
    164–177
assessment of family, 166–168,
    170–171
barriers to, 165–166
elder approval of, 175–176
family as primary client, 176
group meetings, 172–174
informal open-house, 169–171
organizational issues, 164–166
prerehabilitation phase, 169–170
support group participation, 171–
    172
support services for, 150–151
Fear of vision loss, 67–68, 243–244
Fletcher, Dr. Donald, 220
Fovea centralis, function of, 88, 93
Frailty
biopsychological factors in, 117–
    120
World Health Organization,
    definition of, 117–119
Framingham Study, 35
Functioning, components of, 134

G

Gender
and aging, 7, 25, 247
life expectancy and disability, 30

Geriatric Depression Scale, 145
Geriatric Education Centers, 202
Geriatric medicine
medical rehabilitation, 120–121
principles of, 43
syndromes in, 122–126
Glare, 87
forms of, 100
Glaucoma, 33, 63–64, 92–93
acute crisis, 93
and African Americans, 60
closed-angle glaucoma, 63, 93
early detection and treatment, 64
open-angle glaucoma, 63, 92–93
prevalence among older people,
    27
signs of, 92, 93
types of, 63
Group meetings, for family mem-
    bers, 172–174

H

Handicap, definition of, 133
Health Interview Survey, on visual
    impairment and elderly people,
    35–36
Health surveys, listing of major sur-
    veys, 35
Health system reimbursement, 217–
    220
Comprehensive Outpatient Re-
    habilitation Facility (CORF), 221
Hopkins model, 220–221
managed care model, 222
Medicaid, 217, 218, 219
Hearing impairment
and activities of daily living, 42
in dual sensory impairment, 242
prevalence among older people, 27
Hemianopsia, from stroke, 66
Hip fracture, 39, 116
causes of, 125
rehabilitation for, 123
Hispanics

in aging population, 7, 60
and diabetic retinopathy, 60
Hopkins model, health system reimbursement, 220–221
Hypertension, prevalence among older people, 27

I

Income
among the aging population, 7–8, 10
and geographic location, 61
and preventive care, 61
Individualized Written Rehabilitation Program, 157, 164
International Classification of Diseases, blindness/low vision classification, 89
International Classification of Functioning and Disability ICIDH-2), 117
Intraocular pressure, mechanism in, 92

J

Jewish Guild for the Blind, 221
Josephine L. Taylor Leadership Institute, 215

L

Laser surgery
for diabetic retinopathy, 64, 92
for glaucoma, 64
for macular degeneration, 94
Learning
procedural learning, 124
styles for different age groups, 127, 141
Lens, function of, 88
Life expectancy
changes over time, 23, 25–26
and disability, 29–30

extension of, 15–16, 23
life span view (1970–1990), 31
longevity and new life stages, 182
of women, 7, 30, 61
Lighthouse International, 214–215, 222
Lighthouse National Survey on Vision Loss, 35, 215–216
Lighthouse National Vision Rehabilitation Network, 222
Lighting, 99–101
and glare, 100
requirements for low vision, 100–101
Linkages, projects based on, 204–206
Lions Vision Research and Rehabilitation Center, 220
Longitudinal studies, adaptation to vision loss, 234
Longitudinal Study on Aging (LSOA), 37
Long-term care, scope of, 139, 141
Low vision, 59, 66–67, 87–90
prevalence among older people, 5
definition of, 59
neural effects, 95–96
optical effects, 94–95
Low vision rehabilitation, 97–105
adaptive training, 99
goals of, 102
lighting requirements, 99–101
low vision devices, 66–67, 98–99
nonoptical aids, 98
rehabilitation team, 101, 104–105
research and development needs, 102–104

M

Macula, function of, 88
Macular degeneration. *See* Age-related macular degeneration
Magnifiers, 98, 99
Managed care

adequacy of care, 11
future needs, 16
Managed care model, vision rehabilitation reimbursement, 222
Meal preparation, 41
Medicaid
   reimbursement levels, 217
   states' role, 12–13, 219
Medical rehabilitation
   and dementia, 124
   for depression, 124–125
   exercise, 120–121
   and hip fractures, 123
   historical view, 112–113
   intervention needs for, 126–127
Medicare
   inadequate access to, 10
   reform needs, 12
Medication use, polypharmacy, 122
Metamorphosia, 95
Middle age, age span of, 6
Middle class, decline of, 15
Mobility. *See* Orientation and mobility (O&M)
Model Reporting Area, 35
Morbidity curve, meaning of, 29
Mortality curve, meaning of, 29
Muscular system
   and aging, 114–115
   muscle fibers, types of, 115

N

National Advocacy Campaign, 72
National Agenda on Vision and
   Aging, 78–79
   goals of, 79
National Aging and Vision Net-
   work, 71–72
National Center for Health Statistics
   1984 Supplement on Aging, 35
National Center for Health Statistics
   Health Interview Survey, 35
National Health Interview Survey
   on Disability, 35, 36

National Health Service Corps, 202
National Institute of Mental Health,
   202
National Society for the Prevention
   of Blindness, 35
National Vision Rehabilitation Co-
   operative, 215, 222
Native Americans, and diabetic reti-
   nopathy, 60
Neural effects, of low vision, 95–96
Neurological functions, and aging,
   116
Neurotransmitters, and depression,
   144–145
Norpramin, 147
Nottingham Adjustment Scale, 232
Nursing home residents
   rate of visual impairment among,
   38, 59
   urinary incontinence among, 126

O

Older Adult Health and Mood
   Questionnaire, 145–146
Older Americans Act, 191–192
   Title I, 9
   Title III, 202
   Title IV, 202
Open-angle glaucoma, nature of, 63,
   92–93
Optical effects, of low vision, 94–95
Orientation and mobility (O&M),
   40, 69–70
Orthopedic impairment, prevalence
   among older people, 27
Outcome measurement, vision re-
   habilitation, 234–239
Out of the Corner of My Eye (Ring-
   gold), 67

P

Pamelor, 147
Parkinson's disease, 116

Partners III Project, 201, 203, 205, 206
Partners Projects, 184, 194, 199, 203
Paxil, 147
Payback period, for rehabilitation services, 44
Physiological changes, as part of aging, 114–116
Polypharmacy, 122
Presbyopia, 115
Preventive care, and income level, 61
Privitization, of vision rehabilitation services, 216
Professional/Consumer Advocacy Council (PCAC), 203
Profiles in Aging and Vision (Orr), 67
Psychosocial factors, 67–69, 134, 141–151
   depression, 142–147
   family issues, 68–69, 149–151
   fear of vision loss, 67–68, 243–244
   quality-of-life issues, 147–149
   research on, 245–247
Public policy, 8–11, 183–206
   age-related legislation, 9
   and aging network, 189
   coalition, benefits of, 197–201
   collaboration/linkages models, 203–206
   and consumer support groups, 214–215
   and developmental disabilities, 189–190
   funding of aging initiatives, 202
   future agenda, 16–18
   local focus, 201–203
   and marginalized status of aging and disabled populations, 186–189
   Medicare and Medicaid, 10
   needs and emphasis for, 11
   past achievements, 8–9
   and population changes, 23–26
   public confidence, 13–14

Social Security system, 7, 8, 14
   trends related to, 215–217
   and vision rehabilitation, 43–46
Pulmonary function, and aging, 114
Pupil, function of, 88

Q

Quality of life, 147–149
   measurement of, 147–148
   two-factor model, 148
   valued activities, 148

R

Refractive errors, 38, 87, 115
Rehabilitation, 69–78, 134–141
   failure, causes of, 135
   goals of, 134
   historical view, 44, 111–112
   inadequacy of services, 44–45
   older versus younger persons, 140–141
   payback period, 44
   principles of, 134–136
   and secondary conditions, 136–137
   steps in practice of, 136–139
   See also Medical rehabilitation; Vision rehabilitation
Rehabilitation Act, Title VII, 48, 70–71, 157, 213
Research
   adaptation to vision loss, 228–234
   on age/gender/ethnic differences, 245–248
   on co-morbidity, 241–243
   experimental designs, 238
   on family caregiving, 239–241
   on fear of vision loss, 243–244
   on low vision rehabilitation, 102–104
   on peer support groups, 244–245
   rehabilitation outcomes, 234–239
Resilience, meaning of, 69

Retina, function of, 88
Retirement, traditional age of, 25
Rusk, Howard, 113

S

Sclera, function of, 88
Secondary conditions, 39–43
  definition of, 39
  examples of, 39–40
  and rehabilitation, 136–137
Second Longitudinal Study on
  Aging, 37
Second Supplement on Aging (SOA
  II), 35
  on visual loss and aging, 37
Setting Limits (Callahan), 187
Social activities, and visually im-
  paired population, 41
Social class, middle class, decline
  of, 15
Social isolation, 42
Social Security, 7, 8, 14
  inadequacy of funds issue, 12
Social support, 157–159
  and adaptation to vision loss, 231
  and depression, 145
State rehabilitation agencies
  homemaker closures, 213
  and Medicaid, 12–13
Strength training, 121
Stress and coping model
  adaptation to vision loss, 230–231
  depression and vision loss, 143–
  144
Stroke, and hemianopsia, 66
Successful Aging (MacArthur Foundation), 109–110
Supplement on Aging (SOA), 36, 39
Supplemental Security Income
  (SSI), 10
Support groups, 69
  for family members, 171–172
  peer support groups, 244–245

T

T'ai Chi
Telemicroscope, 99
Telescopic systems, 98

U

Urinary incontinence, 125–126

V

Varicose veins, prevalence among
  older people, 27
Vision examination
  goals of, 97
  patient/practitioner interaction,
  96–97
  prescribing, 97–98
Vision rehabilitation, 43–46
  advocacy skills addressed in, 75–
  76
  aging network, role in, 79–80
  barriers to services, 77–78
  certification of practitioners, 218
  and client self-determination, 165
  as community-based service, 76
  and family. *See* Family-oriented
  rehabilitation
  future needs for, 47–49, 72
  health system payment for, 217–
  220
  historical development of, 45, 70–
  72, 217–218
  individualized treatment plan,
  157, 164
  long-term care, 139, 141
  low vision rehabilitation, 97–105
  organizational issues, 165–166
  outcome domains of, 47
  outcomes, research on, 234
  psychosocial factors, 141–151
  referral needs, 73–74

and resilience, 69
skills focused on, 41, 69–70
types of services, 45
vocational rehabilitation, 74–75
Visual conditions
  and activities of daily living, 40, 42
  age-related macular degeneration, 62–63, 93–94
  cataracts, 65–66, 91
  diabetic retinopathy, 64–65, 91–92
  glaucoma, 63–64, 92–93
  low vision, 59, 66–67, 87–90
  stroke-related, 66
  See also Aging and visual impairment
Visual Functioning Questionnaire, 232

Vocational rehabilitation, 111–112
  visual, 74–75

W

Warren, Marjory, 112
Wet-type, age-related macular degeneration, 93
Women
  aging and status of, 25
  as caregivers, 193
  life expectancy, 7, 30, 61
World Health Organization (WHO), 117, 119
World Through Their Eyes (Fangmeier), 67

Z

Zoloft, 147